Talking
To Your
KIDS About
Sex

Talking
To Your
KIDS About
Sex

Mark Laaser, Ph.D.

WATERBROOK
PRESS

Talking to Your Kids About Sex
Published by WaterBrook Press
12265 Oracle Boulevard, Suite 200
Colorado Springs, Colorado 80921

ISBN 978-1-57856-199-5

Library of Congress Cataloging-in-Publication Data
Laaser, Mark R.
    Talking to your kids about sex / Mark Laaser. — 1st ed.
        p.   cm.
    ISBN 1-57856-199-X
        1. Sex—Religious aspects—Christianity.   2. Sex instruction for
children—Religious aspects—Christianity.   3. Child rearing—
Religious aspects—Christianity.   I. Title.
BT708.L32   1999
241'.66—dc21   99-26336
            CIP

Printed in the United States of America
2009

10 9 8 7

To Deb, Sarah, Jon, and Ben
—my family—
practitioners of what I preach.

Contents

Acknowledgments

Writing a book, for me, is always a collaborative effort. Even though I am the one responsible for the words, many people have helped. Whenever I've written a book, someone has encouraged me to do it. In the case of this book, it has not been one person but the voices of many men and women I have worked with around the world. These parents, collectively, have said that someone needs to tell us how to talk to our kids about sex; it might as well be you. My resistance to doing so was high. The subject came up so often, however, that I gave in. Thanks—I think—to all of you out there who bugged me to write what I know.

Writing is also an emotionally and spiritually draining task for me. I could not have taken the time and energy to write this book without the patience of my family during all the time it has taken me away from them. Our computer is also in our TV room, so this patience has involved other sacrifices.

The biggest thanks goes to my wife, Deb. For twenty-six years now, she has been my companion in the journey of marriage, and for twenty-two years in the learning experience of parenting. She has lived with my many sins and mistakes over the years and is a constant reminder of God's grace in my life. She often challenges me in my thinking, and that is a gift. Most of all, she is my practice partner as we seek to understand together what healthy sexuality is all about.

My children, Sarah, Jon, and Ben, have been wondering what I was going to say in this book and whether or not they have heard most of it already. It is a scary thought that there are those who really do know if a father is practicing what he is preaching. I thank them for being my children and for allowing me to practice on them.

There are many professional colleagues to thank for their input on the biblical and psychological points of this book. Dr. Patrick Carnes helped me to formulate much of my early ideas. Eli Machen has been doing workshops with me for years. I can't count the number of hours we have spent talking about being fathers. More than anything, he is a good friend who often reminds me of what is really important. There have been young fathers, like Rob Jackson, who works with me at the Oasis Ministry of the Christian Alliance for Sexual Recovery, who have given me insights about theological and biblical principles. Another is Neal Clement whom I have worked with in the ministry he started to help sex addicts.

Many other men, friends and colleagues in ministry, have challenged my thinking. Among them are Chris Charleton, Jerry Caspel, and Nils Friberg. There are also hundreds of men who must remain nameless—men I have worked with over the years who have given me so much as they have sought to heal.

Then there are those female colleagues, Christian therapists, who have given me much insight into the female perspective of all of this. Ginger Manley has been a friend for years and is the source of the healthy sexuality model I use. Marnie Feree has developed a ministry for women struggling with sexual sin. Marnie and I have spent hours talking about parenting and healthy sexuality. Most of all I thank her for the honesty of all the stories she has told me. Angela Thompson has also shared of herself in this way. Lynn Wildmon, who has worked with me in a ministry for the wives of sex addicts, has also shared of herself and her own journey. Like the men, there are countless women who must remain nameless who have shared their stories with me in workshops over the past few years.

I thank the good people at WaterBrook Press who have had the courage to take on a book like this and for their skills in publishing. Thanks to my agent, Sara Fortenberry, for connecting us. WaterBrook had the wisdom to assign Traci Mullins to this project, an editor who has been wonderful to work with. She has been a tough, insightful, yet gentle friend. Without her, this book wouldn't be finished. Thanks, Traci, for helping me through the adolescence of my own writing.

There were nights when I was tempted to click the delete button and give up on this whole project. Thanks to all of you who have been praying for this book. If it is helpful to any of you, it is because God has been in control. To him be the glory!

A Challenging Task

> The fear of the LORD is the beginning of knowledge, but fools despise wisdom and discipline. Listen, my son, to your father's instruction and do not forsake your mother's teaching. They will be a garland to grace your head and a chain to adorn your neck. My son, if sinners entice you, do not give in to them.
>
> (PROVERBS 1:7-10)

When Solomon wrote these proverbs, he assumed that parents were talking to their children, giving them instruction. And certainly most parents were, and are, trying their best to steer their kids toward wisdom and the fear of the Lord. Solomon would be sadly mistaken, however, if he were assuming that all mothers and fathers are talking to their children about sex and teaching them about God's design for healthy sexuality.

Most parents raising children today would agree that sexuality should be taught at home rather than simply being left to their children's schoolteachers, peers, or popular culture. However, even parents with the best intentions to educate their children about sexuality and the Christian values they cherish are sometimes at a loss as to where to start, how much to talk about, and how often to talk.

Even more perplexing to many parents is the challenge of modeling to their kids healthy sexuality in their own lives and relationships. Most adults in this fallen world have sexual dysfunctions and relational struggles of their own that defy simple solutions. How are they to teach their children about ideals they may not have achieved themselves?

Most important, what does God want their kids to know about sexuality? What should parents say to their kids about issues that have become extremely complex and controversial in our contemporary society?

Talking to children about sex is a frightening task. Not very many parents feel comfortable doing it. There is something about sexuality that is embarrassing and difficult to talk about intimately. It is more likely that we will talk about sex in teasing or joking ways. Genesis 3:6 describes the bite out of the apple that constitutes original sin. The first consequence of that sin is that Adam and Eve recognize they are naked, and they feel ashamed. In other words, one of the consequences of original sin is sexual shame. It is part of our nature since the Fall to have difficulty talking about sex.

I believe, however, that the greatest enemy of sexual wholeness is silence. Silence is one of the tools that Satan uses to prevent people from making healthy sexual choices. When I was growing up in the 1950s and '60s, my parents didn't talk to me about sex except for the traditional mechanical disclosure from my father that came several years after I already knew about the biology of sex. None of my friends were hearing about sex from their parents either. None of us knew enough about sex to talk intelligently or maturely to each other. Even if we did, we were too embarrassed to have an honest discussion. We certainly wouldn't have thought about talking to girls about sex.

When we went to church, it was the same. I do remember one high-school youth group meeting when the girls were taken off to one room and the boys to another. Rather than the pastor talking to us, a medical doctor was brought in. He described to us in great detail every sexually transmitted disease he could think of. I guess he hoped to scare us away from even thinking about being sexual. Of course, most of us boys were already preoccupied with sex. We wondered about girls in general, and cloistering them off in a separate room only increased the mystery.

Finally, in my senior year of high school, we did get "sex education." Anatomy and physiology were explained. The main lesson I remember is that we were supposed to use a condom, and we were to take special care to unroll it right. Again, the girls were taken off into a separate room and shown a film on childbirth. I assumed that it was too painful for the boys to watch. It was the mysterious realm of females to be concerned about such things.

How I longed to talk to someone about the many overwhelming sexual feelings I was having. When I was eleven years old, I discovered that there *was* a source of information. A friend of mine bicycled over to my house on a hot summer day, eyes wide with the joy of discovery. He told me that I just *had* to follow him to a local drugstore. I was skeptical and it was hot, but he persisted.

What he showed me, hidden in a wooden cabinet next to the magazine rack, was a stack of the fattest magazines I had ever seen. I watched in utter terror as he stole one of those magazines. Back in the privacy of my garage, together we unfolded the first picture of a naked female I had ever seen. The woman actually seemed to be smiling at me. At once my brain was flooded with a mixture of fear, excitement, and sexual pleasure. It was a feeling I had never had before, one that I would pursue well into my adult years.

That same magazine also provided us with "advice." There were regular columns and letters about sexual experiences. We were like sponges soaking in the frank discussions about sexuality. We didn't know it then, but we were learning massive amounts of incorrect information about healthy sexuality. Even the cartoons in that magazine, which appealed to my childlike curiosity, were teaching me moral lessons that I didn't question for years to come.

Later that same summer at church camp, the head counselor gathered all of us around a campfire. He instructed us to write our main sin on a piece of paper. Without hesitation I wrote *Playboy* magazine. He said that if we were willing to give up this sin, we should throw our paper on the fire, and God would consume it. What a relief that was! What a disappointment one week later when, back home, I hopped on my bicycle and it headed for that same drugstore. How mad and disappointed I was with God. For the next twenty-five years I struggled to break free from the pull of an addiction to pornography and other sexual sins.

Can you imagine what it might have been like if that night at the dinner table, when my father asked me, "How was your day?" I could have said, "Dad, I'm glad you asked that question because I'd like to discuss with you the information I read about sex today in this magazine." I wonder what my reaction would have been if my mother had said to me one day, "Mark, I know you've been looking at those magazines in the garage. I'm not mad at you. I think it's normal for you to be curious about sex. I would like to talk to you about what women are really like and what healthy sexuality means to them."

My parents did the best they knew how to do. I don't blame them for their lack of instruction. I'm sure that no one talked to them much about sex when they were kids. As parents, they probably weren't talking to other parents either. When they were young parents, information about sexuality was nonexistent. Masters and Johnson hadn't even met yet. There certainly weren't any Christian materials available.

The sexual revolution that started in the 1960s has had many sinful consequences. On the other hand, our culture's attempt to remove some of the shame surrounding sex has led to much more open and honest conversations. Of course, there is much to be ashamed about in our current sexual culture. We should not forget, however, that God made us male and female and that sex is his way of allowing us to participate in the joy of creation. Sexual shame and embarrassment is a problem if it prevents us from communicating with each other the fact that sex is a God-given and joyful experience between a husband and wife.

A healthy understanding of sexuality is not taught to children during one perfunctory conversation about "the birds and the bees." Rather, parents are presented with "teachable moments" at every stage of a child's development. My goal is to prepare you to have a lifetime of effective, age-appropriate conversations with your kids about sex by outlining the information they need at various ages and how you can provide it in loving and spiritually mature ways.

Chapters 4–8 of this book will walk you through the typical developmental issues children face at various ages and outline for you what I believe your tasks are as you guide your children's healthy sexual development from birth into their early adult years. I realize that by the time you read this book your kids may already have passed through some of the developmental stages I identify. Please don't feel that it's ever too late to teach your children about healthy sexuality. There is no magical cutoff beyond which it is too late for us to move closer to God's design; sexuality is something we learn about throughout life. So if your kids are already in the thick of things in terms of their sexual development, don't be intimidated or discouraged. Use the principles I describe to engage in the kind of conversation that will continue for a lifetime. This can even mean going back and having conversations about the material regarding earlier stages.

Also be aware that the age ranges identified are based on generally accepted divisions but that children grow physically, emotionally, and spiritually at different rates. The information that is appropriate for most at a particular time may not be appropriate for others. It is up to you to decide if your child is ready for certain kinds of information.

Chapter 2 describes a model of healthy sexuality that I have found particularly useful through the years, and most of what I suggest in this book builds on its assumptions. I trust you will find it biblical and balanced. I am aware that, given the clinical work I have done over the years, I may have placed too much emphasis on describing issues in terms of problems that can develop. I don't want to scare you; I simply want you to take these issues seriously so that you will be a loving resource for your children.

Chapter 3 suggests several principles of productive communication and healthy conversation. I hope it will both help you feel better equipped as you begin to talk to your children about sex and remind you of basic communication skills that are essential throughout your children's lives.

Last, but not least, the first chapter of this book, one of the most challenging but also one of the most important, will help you explore some of your personal issues so you can become whole as a man or woman and, if you are married, more intimate as a couple. It will also help you to practice talking to your spouse or a trusted friend about the sexual issues that might be interfering with your ability to talk to your children openly and effectively about sex. My counseling with individuals and couples has convinced me that difficulties related to sexuality (in a broad sense of the term) underlie many of our troubles in relating to God, to ourselves, and to others. The more healthy you are in your own sexuality, the more prepared you will be to help your children develop into the men and women God has designed them to be.

This book does not attempt to give you all the medical or scientific information about sexuality you will need. There are no diagrams, no explicit biological sexual information. Other books, including some written from a Christian perspective, explain and illustrate anatomy, physiology, and human sexual response. We are the inheritors of a generation of research that has dispelled many harmful myths and offered healing for many sexual dysfunctions. We can benefit from that information as long as we understand that it is to be used in the context of marriage. In the resource section at the end of this book, I have listed several books that you may find useful as you attempt to teach your children what they need to know and as you explore your own sexual issues.

My own sexual shame, much of it left over from my sinful past, tells me that I shouldn't be writing a book about this topic. One of my fears is that others will look at my children to see if they are examples of what their father is trying to teach. So, like Daniel, it seems that I may be entering the lions' den. I pray that you, the reader, will accept that I have learned from my own mistakes much of what I have to say. What compels me to write are the voices of the hundreds of men and women I have worked with over the past fifteen years who suffer the consequences of sexual sin. All of them can trace problems with their sexuality back to childhood. Without exception, they say they long to have talked more to their parents about sex when they were growing up.

I believe in spiritual warfare. I believe that Satan doesn't want us talking about this topic. As you read this book in an attempt to become a better parent, beware of that inner voice telling you to be silent, to not embarrass yourself, to not raise topics you really don't want to get into. Beware, also, of those sexual demons from your own past telling you to keep your own secrets, that you have no business trying to teach your kids about healthy sexuality because your own failures disqualify you. The truth is, one of the greatest gifts you can give your child is a willingness to talk, even about your own sexual sins and questions. Just as I must disregard those voices that tell me I must be a perfect communicator in order to write a perfect book, I ask you to disregard those voices that will tell you that you must be a perfect parent if you want to teach your children about their God-given sexuality.

I pray that this book will be a helpful resource for you, one that will lead to loving relationships between you and your children. As much as I hope and pray that my own interpretation of God's design and of biblical truth has been guided by the Holy Spirit, I also pray that as you read it you will be similarly inspired by God's loving presence in your life. May you find in these pages what you need to prepare yourself to educate your children and model for them the beauty of what God has ordained for human beings to cherish and enjoy.

CHAPTER ONE

Preparing to Talk Effectively

Bill and Barbara were the proud parents of a thirteen-year-old son and a fifteen-year-old daughter. Before they even met, they had dated many others in an attempt to find that "right" person. None of this had been all that dramatic. Growing up in a permissive culture, however, had influenced them early on about sexual "tolerance." While both Bill and Barbara were rather normal teenagers, they had both experienced sexual intercourse with other partners before meeting each other. Bill, in fact, had been with several sexual partners. When they met each other, they fell in love and felt that it would be hurtful to tell each other about their earlier sexual experiences. They felt shame, but thought that what the other person didn't know wouldn't hurt them.

In the early years of their marriage, Bill and Barbara enjoyed a good sexual relationship. When through the discipleship of another young couple they became Christians, their guilt about past sexual experiences bothered both of them. They believed, however, that they would always be faithful to each other. So once again, silently, they decided to keep their secrets and not risk hurting each other with the truth.

As the stresses of children, careers, and money squeezed them, they found that they didn't take as much time for their relationship. Their sexual relationship suffered. Bill began to be resentful about the frequency of their sexual encounters but didn't feel comfortable talking to Barbara about his feelings. More and more he found himself being tempted by other women. He didn't know what to do with those feelings. He also began looking at pornography. He justified this by thinking that he needed some sexual excite-

ment in his life. Bill even considered showing it to Barbara; maybe it would spice up their relationship.

Bill and Barbara's daughter began dating a boy three years her senior. Both Bill and Barbara wanted to talk to her about their concerns, but since they had never talked to her about romantic relationships in general, they didn't know how to begin the conversation. One day, Barbara discovered a pornographic magazine in their son's bedroom. When she told Bill about it, she expected him to have a talk with their son. Bill found that the thought of doing so brought up such feelings of shame and guilt that he didn't know what to say.

Bill and Barbara are typical of more Christian couples than we might think. Their failure to talk honestly about their own sexual history and feelings left both of them with deep-seated sexual shame and produced an ongoing silence in their family about sexual issues. This silence will have potentially devastating effects on their marriage and on their children, who may not get appropriate information or moral guidance about their own sexual development.

One of the main reasons parents don't talk to their children about sex is that they are uncomfortable discussing the topic themselves. Because modeling a healthy relationship between men and women is every bit as important as the actual conversations we have with our kids about sex, the first task we must approach as parents is exploring and discussing our own beliefs and feelings about the subject. This chapter is designed to help you feel more comfortable talking to each other about sex.

I realize that this is a challenging task, and for some of you a potential hornet's nest of difficult issues. Before your own fears and frustrations cause you to put this book down and neglect to teach your children about issues you yourself find difficult, please let me offer some words of encouragement. As I have dealt with my own sexual issues and helped other individuals and parents to do the same, I have become convinced that God is lovingly in control of each of our journeys, if we let him be in control. He will not let issues come up for you without also providing you with resources to deal with them. As you face the possibility that the task of exploring your own sexual beliefs and experiences is a potentially painful one, I would like for you to consider that, if you choose to take it, you will be doing so for the benefit of your children. Your willingness to grow in your own sexual wholeness can be a tremendous gift to both your spouse and your kids.

BEYOND THE BIRDS AND THE BEES

At some point in their children's lives, many parents gather up their courage and find a way to present some of the basic facts of sexuality and reproduction. However, my personal and professional experience leads me to believe that most parents say too little, too late. Even if they do successfully transmit information about the biology of sex, most parents don't realize how crucial it is to take the conversation to the next level. Our children need to know about much more than where babies come from and how to avoid having babies themselves. I believe that one of our primary tasks as parents is to teach and model healthy male/female relationships and to create a vision in our children's minds and hearts for the rich, fully developed relationship that married couples can enjoy.

One of the best ways to teach and model is to talk to our children as a couple, not just as individual parents. But how are we supposed to talk to our children as a couple about sex if we haven't talked to each other about it? Single parents, or those married to someone other than their child's biological parent, must also become comfortable talking about their experiences, beliefs, and feelings regarding sexuality.

In this chapter I suggest several different ways to work toward greater personal wholeness, a healthier and more loving marriage, and deeper confidence in talking to your kids about the whole gamut of sexual development. Some of you will already have done much of this work; others will be just getting started. If the issues and exercises presented in this chapter seem intimidating, I understand. Fully preparing yourself to talk to your kids about healthy sexuality is not an easy task.

Please don't make the mistake of thinking that you can't have any effective conversations with your kids until you have successfully completed all the tasks I suggest. No parent will ever be perfect, no matter how much personal work he or she does. Becoming sexually whole is a long process for most of us. You may find that some of the issues that come up for you during the process of exploring your own sexuality will need to be deferred to a later time. You may come back to this chapter many times, even after you have read the whole book and begun implementing some of its suggestions in conversations with your children. Please don't feel that you have to complete every exercise in this chapter and become a shining model of healthy sexuality before you can parent effectively. If that were true, none of us would have a chance! So take the material in this chapter seriously, but relax. Deal with your own issues at your own pace, and let your spouse do the same.

Another common mistake people make is thinking that they can or should handle all problems by themselves. You may find that you need some help individually or as a couple to process various feelings effectively. In the resource section at the back of this book, you will find some telephone numbers of national organizations to call for help. Counselors at these numbers will be able to strategize with you about the kind of help you may need and how to get it.

You may also want to ask your pastor or trusted church leaders for help or a referral to a qualified counselor. I know that not everyone has the necessary financial resources to afford extensive professional counseling, but many Christian counselors will work for reduced fees. Many pastors are capable of working with you as well. There also may be other couples in your church who have lived through things you're going through and who would be willing to share their experience.

Finally, I have observed that one of the deadliest devices Satan uses to destroy couples is the phenomenon of blame. When issues come up for you as a couple, are you willing to look at your own responsibility? This is not always easy to do, I know. Your spouse may be doing things wrong, but can you avoid placing blame and instead focus on getting through whatever problem comes up? Being able to look honestly at yourself is important, but this does not mean that you should blame yourself either. Couples who successfully resolve problems are those who can both take responsibility for their behavior and seek to grow emotionally and spiritually. As you read and begin to talk to each other about sexual and relational issues, consider saying this prayer together:

"God, we seek to be faithful parents to our children and to provide them with the best upbringing we can. We want our home to be a safe home. And as our children grow, we want them to learn about many things including your gift of healthy sexuality. Help us know how to both model this and instruct them about how you would have them embrace this gift. Guard and direct our conversations with each other. Please help us as a couple to grow in our spiritual and emotional relationship. Also, if there are sexual wounds in our relationship and in our past that need healing, please direct us in our journey to find that healing. Amen."

A NOTE TO SINGLE OR REMARRIED PARENTS

Don't close this book if you are a single parent! If you are divorced or widowed, or if you are currently married but not to the biological parent of your child, don't be discouraged by the emphasis that this book places on couples. You still can and should complete the exercises I suggest. I would simply advise you to do them and talk about them with a trusted friend or your current spouse. Or consider finding several single parents to study this book together. A group of your peers can provide you with critical support and help you put some of these principles into practice.

If you are divorced and have a civil relationship with your former spouse, you might even be bold enough to do this work with him or her.

You may need to have a counselor present. I strongly encourage you to at least come to some common understanding and mutual decisions about what you and your former spouse are teaching your children about sex (as well as other moral truth). You owe it to your children to try to do this. I am fully aware that, for some divorced parents, this kind of cooperation is not possible. If you are remarried and raising children, you will want to have these discussions with your current spouse. It is a sacred responsibility for two adults living under the same roof with children to be of like mind in providing them with safety, modeling, and instruction.

If you are not remarried and are living alone, you can still do a wonderful job of teaching your kids about healthy sexuality. While it is good for a child to hear about sexuality from both a man and woman at the same time, that is not always possible, even for married couples.

One myth we need to dispel is that only a woman can talk to a female child and only a man can talk to a male child. Some of the most wonderful conversations take place between a mother and her son or between a father and his daughter. Such conversations illustrate that men and women don't need to be a mystery to each other and that, in many ways, our sexual needs are not that different. Establishing a pattern of talking freely with any of your children on any subject will serve you well as they mature and will enable you to have a series of ongoing, productive conversations.

You will find that most teachable moments about sexuality, even for married couples, arise when one parent is alone with a child. Of course, at other times you may correctly sense, "My son needs to talk to a man about that" or "My daughter needs to talk to a woman about this." Same-sex perspective can sometimes help a child, especially adolescents and teenagers, feel more comfortable.

You may find it helpful to find a person of the opposite sex, someone with whom you have a mature and nonsexual relationship, to serve as a role model and guide for your child. Your parents, pastor, church elders, and your child's coaches or teachers may be excellent candidates. I have known many people whose most positive memories of talking about sex go back to a special person in their lives who took the time to talk to them about a specific sexual topic.

In sharing with this role model the responsibility for imparting healthy attitudes to your child, you may want to participate with the two of them in a conversation on healthy sexuality. You'll want to talk to this person before talking to your kids so you can review what you will say.

I would encourage you to read through all the chapters in this book, knowing that you will be the one who will have most of the conversations with your child and that you want to be well equipped. You can even be creative by asking yourself, "How would a father (or mother) handle this?" There is no reason you cannot be the best resource for your child. Be of good courage and be gentle with yourself. You'll do fine.

WHY DON'T WE TALK TO EACH OTHER?

Difficulty talking to each other about sex can be caused by a few problems common to many people. First, as a couple you may have a variety of sexual difficulties. Second, you may have a sexual history that causes you to be ashamed of who you are sexually. As difficult as these things are to talk about, my personal and professional experience has convinced me that we will be much better models to our kids if we learn how to communicate about these issues. While this is not a book that seeks to explain technical sexual problems, my suggestions about how to have initial conversations about them can begin directing you toward the help you may need in order to heal.

Sexual Difficulties

Paul and Andrea are like many couples. When they were dating, everything seemed pretty exciting. They waited for marriage to consummate their sexual relationship. On the honeymoon things went pretty well. Several months later, however, as they adjusted to the routine of jobs and daily schedules, they had less time for each other. Paul noticed that Andrea seemed less interested in sex and that he had to ask in more convincing ways. Frequency was becoming less and less, and Paul was getting angry about it. When they did have sex, Andrea seemed less than enthusiastic.

Both of them worried that something was wrong with them. They believed a common myth that if sex is not always good, the marriage is going bad. Paul didn't know how to tell Andrea about his frustrations, and Andrea was becoming more and more afraid of him. The more afraid she got, the more she shut down sexually. This vicious cycle persisted until sex was virtually absent in their relationship.

Paul and Andrea's problems are rather common and certainly not impossible to talk about and heal. Given the many jokes that are told by comedians and others about sexuality and marriage, it is easy to surmise that many marriages suffer from some kind of sexual difficulty. Following are a few of the most common ones.

Frequency. All experts agree that there is no "normal" amount of sexual activity between couples. Couples vary from being sexual several times a day to several times a year—or not at all. Frequency may depend on the age of the couple, how long they have been married, and a variety of other factors. The difficulty arises when one partner would like to be sexual more often than the other.

Our current culture gives us rather false expectations about how often a couple should be sexual. Given the titles of many articles on magazine covers at our grocery stores, one might be tempted to think that for healthy couples sex takes place all the time. Those of us who have had problems with pornography will have totally unrealistic expectations about sexual frequency. The key is to talk about it and to respect and honor each other. Having frequent sex is not necessarily a sign of a healthy marriage.

Different sexual likes and dislikes. Many couples simply don't talk at all about what they like sexually or what really gives them pleasure. When they do, sometimes they can't agree on the nature of sexual activity. One partner may want to engage in sexual activities that the other doesn't like or is even repulsed by. One partner may even think and say to the other partner, "If you really loved me, you would do this." Some partners accuse their spouses of not being spontaneous or playful enough. I have even heard many Christians argue about whether or not certain sexual activities are "biblical." As awkward as it may be for some couples, talking honestly about what each enjoys and feels comfortable with is critical to a healthy sexual relationship.

Sexual dysfunction. Most couples experience some form of sexual dysfunction at one time or another. This simply means that normal sexual response has somehow broken down, dysfunctioned. One of the most common problems for men is impotence. This can be caused by either physical or emotional factors. Another common problem for men is premature ejaculation. Some women have problems with self-lubricating, painful intercourse, or an inability to experience orgasm. These common problems can be overcome with the help of medical doctors or Christian counselors who specialize in treating the physical or emotional roots of these dysfunctions.

Sexual Wounds

Talking to your spouse or anyone else about sex may be difficult if past sexual wounds have damaged your spirit and created sexual shame.

Ann was sexually molested by an older neighbor boy when she was a young girl. When she was twelve, her older brother talked her into being sexual with him several times. In high school, Ann was sexually active with several boyfriends.

When she met her husband, Bob, she fell in love with him but was not able to tell him about her sexual abuse or any of her sexual history. Both Bob and Ann committed to being sexually abstinent before marriage. Ann thought about sex often, however, and it seemed to her that it was harder for her to wait for sex than it was for Bob. Occasionally, she flirted with other young men and found herself fantasizing about being sexual with them.

When they did get married, Ann enjoyed sex and was always available for it. She was even rather aggressive about initiating sex. When she did this, Bob often seemed disinterested. Ann wondered if there was something wrong with her but didn't have anyone to talk to about it. She found herself reading many women's magazines about how to make sex in marriage more exciting. Bob found himself feeling inadequate as a man since he didn't seem able to satisfy Ann.

Ann has no idea that her past sexual wounds and history are profoundly affecting her. If Bob and Ann are to get help, she will need to tell him about her history and get some healing from it. Ann experiences a lot of sexual shame that will hurt her in trying to be honest with Bob. Several kinds of sexual shame can arise from our past experiences.

Discomfort with who we are physically. Almost all of us go through periods of our development when we don't like how we look. Most of us have stories about thinking we were unattractive. Many of us were teased by others about various parts of our bodies. Some of us were too short, tall, fat, or thin. Some of us have other physical characteristics that even now we don't like. Admitting this to our partner can be a freeing experience. We will usually find out that these things don't bother our partner at all, or at least not as much as they bother us.

Sexual trauma. Second Samuel 13:1-32 recounts the tragic story of David's daughter, Tamar. I doubt that many of us have ever heard a sermon preached about Tamar's brother Amnon sexually molesting her. The consequences to Tamar were devastating, but she was told not to even talk about it: "Her brother Absalom said to her, 'Has that Amnon, your brother, been with you? Be quiet now, my sister; he is your brother. Don't take this thing to heart.' And Tamar lived in her brother Absalom's house, a desolate woman" (2 Samuel 13:20).

My advice to the contrary is, *do* take these things to heart and *do* talk about them. Estimates vary but have generally held that one-third of all women and one-fourth of all men have experienced some form of sexual trauma. Some people don't remember their sexual abuse; it may have been so powerful that their brain has blocked out the memories.

Sexual dysfunction or problems, as described above, may be the result of remembered or repressed sexual trauma. Resources listed at the end of this book can help victims identify and begin to heal from this damage. Although healing may be a long journey, there is lots of hope. The path to healing begins with talking about the trauma with trusted people, counselors, pastors, and one's spouse.

Sexual history. As Christians we value being virgins when we get married. When this is not the case, the history of our prior sexual experience can be painful to share. This can also be true for those who remarry after the death of a spouse or after a divorce. While it is not necessary or advisable to discuss the graphic details of past sexual activity, I do believe that it is a freeing experience to share sexual histories as much as possible. To not do so is to always wonder what one's spouse would think if he or she knew. This can have an inhibiting effect on sexual conversation in the future.

Sexual addiction. Sexual addiction is like any addiction: It simply means that a person can't stop engaging in various forms of sexual sin. Sex addicts involve themselves in an ever-increasing pattern of out-of-control sexual behavior. They confuse sex with their need to be loved and may be aggressive in their pursuit of sexual activity. Their brain chemistry even gets "hooked" on a certain amount of sex, and they need to experience it just as alcoholics need to drink to achieve the same feeling of a "high." Sex addicts can even be addicted to sex in their marriages, thinking that if sex is frequent and exciting their problems will be solved. This belief can create unbelievable tension in a marriage.

Even more devastating, however, is the tremendous pain that sex outside the marriage can create. Even acting out sexual fantasy through pornography and/or masturbating can be disastrous. Sex addiction will shut down healthy communication in a marriage faster than anything else.

There is much hope for healing for sex addicts and their spouses.

Sex addicts, however, can't heal themselves. A Christian counselor who is experienced in treating sex addiction must be consulted. Again, several helpful resources are listed in the back of this book.

Incest. This is the most painful topic to raise. Sexual communication in a marriage will be completely destroyed if one of the partners is committing incest with one of the children. The vast majority of incest perpetrators are themselves victims of some form of sexual abuse. It is vital that a family who experiences this gets the help they need.

Usually, incest must be reported to local authorities. The results of this will vary depending on the current age of the victim and the nature of the sexual activity. Jail time for the perpetrator is possible. I cannot advise strongly enough that even in the face of undeniable consequences, this situation must be talked about. The Bible is very harsh with those who harm children. However, I have known many families who have healed from these devastating wounds and are still together. The key, as with everything else, is to be honest and to talk.

HEALING CONVERSATION

Ann and Bob began to think about having children. Somewhere in her spirit, Ann knew that she and Bob needed to start talking about sex. Ann knew that she could get pregnant, but she didn't want the sexual tensions in their marriage to affect how they parented. So she took the courageous first step. Ann went to her pastor and told him about her concerns. The pastor referred Ann to a female Christian therapist who had experience treating sexual trauma. Ann finally told someone else about the secret of her sexual abuse. She started going to a group for women who had been sexually abused and began to face her sexual shame and how it had manifested itself in her life.

Ann's therapist helped her prepare to tell Bob her story. They scheduled an appointment together, during which Ann told Bob about her past sexual abuse. Ann was extremely anxious about how he would react and was amazed to find that he was sup-

portive and extremely caring. As Bob heard the story, he was naturally angry about the abuse and hurt by some aspects of the history. He was also relieved because hearing the story put into perspective some things about his marriage.

Bob found that he could talk to his pastor about his feelings, and the two of them scheduled regular meetings. This pastor allowed Bob to be angry and simply listened and affirmed his feelings. Ann's therapist also began to work with both Ann and Bob as a couple. For the first time in their marriage, they began to learn how to talk to each other. Their pastor also met with them several times and directed how they might have quiet times of prayer and Bible study together. The therapist invited them to participate in a group of couples who were also dealing with issues of sexual growth. This group met weekly to pray, study Scripture, and talk about sex.

After several months of steady emotional and spiritual growth, Ann and Bob began working on their sexual relationship with their therapist. Issues of frequency and practice were now much easier to talk about. Ann went through several phases of growth. When she was first allowed to talk about her sexual abuse, she found that she went through a period in which she did not want to be sexual at all. Later, she also realized that being sexual was one of the ways she thought she received affirmation from men. At times her sexual fantasies were really about being loved. Because of her sexual abuse, she was uncomfortable with several kinds of sexual touching. Since she and Bob were now able to talk about these, they were able to adjust and grow together. Bob was able to tell Ann how inadequate he had felt in being able to please her.

Gradually, Bob and Ann found that the emotional and spiritual nature of their relationship was much more important than sex. They now have a regular therapy resource to help them through the rough times. Their pastor is providing spiritual direction for them. They belong to an accountability group of other couples. They have learned new ways of talking and have talked to each other about things they never imagined putting out on the table. If they are able to have children, they will be wonderfully prepared to talk to them about sex.

I use Bob and Ann's example because their story of sexual trauma illustrates that even the roughest of issues can be dealt with successfully. The key is that both Bob and Ann were willing to work on their own issues. Ultimately they both sought counsel and safe places to express their feelings. They could not have done this by themselves.

You will also notice how much courage it took for Ann to initiate this process of growth. Her history caused her serious sexual shame. Out of love for her husband and possible future children, however, she was able to face her feelings and overcome her shame. Sometimes it is hardest to be honest with those we love the most. We may be afraid that they will leave us when they hear our whole story. Ann talked to "safe" people—first her pastor, then her therapist. Even if you think that you don't have the financial means to get professional help, don't give up on finding a safe person with whom you can talk.

The first thing I suggest as preparation for a healthy dialogue with your spouse, counselor, pastor, or friend is extensive personal reflection. It is difficult to share thoroughly and honestly with another person before you have been honest with yourself and identified the issues and experiences that have contributed to your views on sexuality.

Sometimes we may not be fully aware of a history that is affecting us. We just know that something isn't right about the way we feel. We may experience depression, anxiety, or other feelings, and not know where they come from. This is a very common phenomenon. Some memories get buried. Some patterns of behavior are so old that we have forgotten where they started. Even if we remember some things, we may not know how to interpret them or how important they are.

If any of this is true for you, probably no amount of personal reflection will help you identify all of the issues you need to deal with. You will need to talk to someone who will encourage you and who can help you know both the right questions to ask of yourself and how to interpret the information you discover.

Now, as you're reading this, take a deep breath. You may be wondering, "Why is this guy telling me to do all of this work? After all, he's a counselor himself. These things are important to him, but isn't it better to just let the past be the past and move on with our lives?" You're right, resolving sexual issues involves a lot of work, and you don't absolutely need to do it. You can still love your children and be good parents. But I have personally seen and experienced the invaluable rewards of greater sexual wholeness and the way it benefits a couple's children. Hopefully you will be convinced of those rewards yourself by the time you finish this book, if you aren't already. Meanwhile, even a small amount of growth on your part can make you feel more prepared to converse with your children about sex. Isn't that worth some effort?

Let's assume that you have done some personal reflection either by yourself or with a counselor, pastor, or friend. Now, for the purpose of finishing the rest of this chapter, I suggest that you find a notebook in which you can feel free to write. Consider this your own "sacred" document. Agree with your spouse that you will not look at these notebooks without each other's permission. Then begin to work through the exercises outlined in the following pages.

Keep in mind that there are several ways to complete these exercises. Some of you will decide to work on them as a couple and will talk about them easily. You will march right through this chapter. If you are highly task-oriented, however, beware of completing these exercises too quickly or superficially. They may take several days or weeks. I suggest that you schedule regular times to talk about what you've written. Establish a contract in which you make appointments with each other and honor those appointments as priorities. Consider getting out of the house and going somewhere else to have your meetings.

Some of you may encounter those painful feelings I've been writing about, and you will need to schedule times with counselors, pastors, or friends to do these exercises. If this is the case, the process may take weeks or months. Don't be discouraged by that. You are not in a race. Remember, you don't have to be perfectly sexually healthy in order to continue talking to your kids about developmental and sexual issues that come up for them as they grow.

On page 31 is a list of rules for having a safe conversation with each other. You may also want to skip to chapter 3 where the principles of having safe conversations with your kids are discussed. All of those principles apply to having healthy conversations with each other. I hope and pray that this book will be the kind of resource you will have to put down at times because it will bring up many things for you to think and pray about.

I once worked with an old German carpenter who taught me many carpentry skills. The most important thing he taught me, however, is that when you get tired or frustrated with a project, stop for a while. There are many crooked or sloppy projects in my house that would indicate I didn't always put this lesson into practice. I have found that patience is a skill that can be acquired with practice. Honor any need you feel to take "time-outs." Come back to these exercises later. Be aware, however, that the flip side of not having enough patience is having too much avoidance. It is one thing to take time to do these exercises carefully. It is another to start and never finish them. If this process is difficult for you, you will be tempted to stall or avoid it altogether. If you experience a lot of resistance, consider asking for more support from your spouse or friends, or get professional help so you can continue to grow, however slowly, for the benefit of your most important relationships. You will be glad you did.

MINING FOR TRUTH

Here are the exercises I have found helpful for couples as they prepare to begin or continue to talk to each other about sexuality. (Remember, the same exercises apply to single parents, too.) As you begin writing your responses to the questions posed in this section, let the sample journal entries from couples who have gone through this process give you direction and encouragement.

Family

I remember how sexually charged the atmosphere always was when Dad was around. When I was a teenager, he seemed to leer at me. And I remember many a meal that ended prematurely when he made off-color jokes that embarrassed Mom. From Dad I think I learned that women are primarily for men to prey on and belittle. And Mom always acted like sex was something dirty.

—SARAH, AGE 36

My grandparents had one of those rare romances that you see in old movies. Well into their eighties, they were still clearly in love. They often told stories about their dating days, and the night before my grandmother suddenly died in her sleep, they were dancing in each other's arms at a local club. I can only hope that someday I will experience the kind of passion and tenderness in a relationship that they enjoyed for over sixty-five years.

—JEFF, AGE 24

1. Your family may or may not have talked about sex. Perhaps one of your parents did and the other didn't. Someone in your family might have actually said, "In our family we don't talk about that." Make a list of all of your immediate family members and ask yourself the question, "What messages did I get from them?" Then next to each name write what you think the message was. For example:

Dad: Always joked about sex. Put Mom down for not being sexual enough. Teased my sisters about their bodies. Asked lots of questions about my sexual "adventures." I found pornography in his closet when I was eleven. He knew I had it, but he never talked about it. He always seemed to emphasize the physical aspects of sex and nothing else.

—ROB, AGE 27

Remember that you can also receive strong messages through silence. If no one ever talks about sex, the obvious message is that sex is bad or evil.

Even someone who never said a word to you directly about sex may have modeled something to you by their silence.

Mom: She never talked to me about sex, but she did worry about what time I came home from dates. She was concerned about something that I assumed was sexual danger. From that, I received the message that sex is dangerous. I might also have assumed that it happened only after midnight because my mom seemed to relax if I was home from dates before then.

—MARK, AGE 48

If you experienced some form of invasive sexual trauma from a family member, note that next to his or her name and describe how you think that affected you. Include the effect you think it has had on your current and/or past marriage. If this becomes too painful, you are not ready for this exercise. Stop what you're doing and consider making an appointment to talk to a professional about your experience.

Brother, Stan: When I was twelve, Stan started coming into my room while I was dressing. I hated it, but he was older and told me to stop being such a prude. He said that older girls liked being watched. Later he started touching me. He finally left for college before he could talk me into intercourse with him. I know that this has profoundly affected how I feel about my husband initiating sex. My mom also knew that this was happening and didn't do anything about it. I have a hard time trusting women with whom I might talk about my sexual fears.

—ALICE, AGE 32

2. From our sexual experiences and the messages we receive about them, we internalize themes about sexuality and ourselves as sexual beings. Make a list of the themes—both positive and negative—you learned from your family. There are thousands of possible themes. Here are some examples:
   • Sex is never to be talked about.
   • Men like sex, women don't.

- Women always need to be on guard against aggressive men.
- Men can't control their sexual desires.
- God intends for sex to take place in marriage.
- I must not be a very attractive person.
- I am an attractive person.
- Good Christian couples don't have sexual problems.
- God helps all those who are willing to work their problems out.
- Sex is a wonderful gift from God.

School

I was so self-conscious when I got to junior high. I had acne and was a little on the chubby side. I was embarrassed by my body. All of the handsome boys at school seemed to get to be with all the girls they wanted.

—JEFF, AGE 40

My health teacher was a really neat person. He seemed to take sex talk seriously and didn't tease about it. He carefully explained things to us and set a great example. Even though he didn't talk in Christian terms, he was a very moral man. He taught us the value of respecting girls and the importance of waiting to be sexual with someone we really loved. He was so manly and gentle at the same time. He seemed to really care. He has been a model to me ever since.

—PETER, AGE 27

Our basketball coach was so respected by everyone, it seemed. Our team was undefeated in the girls' AA division. I wonder what people would have thought if they knew how he came on to some of us at practice. He gave me the creeps.

—TAMARA, AGE 29

3. What was the nature of sex education at your school? What courses or instruction did you have?
4. Recall sexuality-related experiences that happened at school. Don't think these have to be dramatic. For example, do you remember comparing

yourself to other kids during physical-education classes? Many of us remember that first public shower after gym class. Record any embarrassment you felt.

5. What sexual messages, spoken or unspoken, did you receive from specific classes or teachers? Write about these messages, received anytime from elementary school through college.

6. Make a list of all the sexual themes you learned at school. Some may be similar to those you learned at home or other places. Remember that a theme can be taught by how things were handled. For example, if boys were taught separately from girls, the theme is that boys and girls can't or shouldn't talk about sex together. Another theme is that girls and boys have "private" information that only they can learn.

Church

One day all of us went over to our youth pastor's house. He had Playboy *magazines there and didn't seem to think anything about it. I was amazed and wanted to look at them but didn't dare.*

—DAVID, AGE 42

Our priest used to always preach about the evils of sex. He said that we all should wait until we were married to have sex, but sex seemed like something dirty when he talked about it. It seemed like we would all go to hell if we simply had a sexual thought.

—ADAM, AGE 27

My Sunday-school teacher took some of us girls out for lunch one day and asked us how it was going with boys. We didn't know what to say. She was very kind and said that she wondered if we had any questions or concerns about sex. She told us a story from her life when she was our age. Some of us began to open up, and we talked for several hours. It was so wonderful to be able to talk to each other and to a safe adult. I will never forget that.

—HANNAH, AGE 33

7. What was the nature of any sex education that you had at church or other religious institutions? Did your youth group ever discuss sexual topics?

8. Have you ever heard any sermons or teachings on sexuality by religious leaders? If so, what impressed you or what have you remembered?

9. What verses of Scripture, if any, strike you as having special sexual meaning? Are there any biblical figures, such as King David, whom you like or dislike because of the sexual examples or messages they portray? If so, write about them and the messages they've given you about sexuality.

10. Have you ever been disappointed by a religious leader who has sinned sexually? If so, write about what this betrayal of trust was like for you.

11. List all the themes about sexuality that you've learned from your church experience and from religious institutions in general. These themes will involve lessons you learned about God's attitude toward sex. For example, you may have been led to believe that God doesn't seem to care much for sex; it is only for procreation. You may have learned that all sexual thinking is bad or dangerous. You might have been taught that women should submit to their husbands even if they don't enjoy sex. Maybe people of faith seemed to be hypocrites, not practicing what they preached. On the other hand, perhaps you have observed wonderful models of marital love and fidelity. Record both positive and negative themes.

Media

My friends were always looking at the teen magazines to see what they should look like. I never had the money to afford all the clothes. My figure was not like those young women either. I tried and tried but could never seem to be like those pictures. I felt almost doomed.

—DEBRA, AGE 26

When I was eleven, my friend showed me a "dirty" magazine he had found. I couldn't believe it. There were things in there I had never seen before. All the women seemed to enjoy sex so much. I learned about practices that I thought were normal. I also got the wrong idea about how women are supposed to look.

—MARTY, AGE 40

All the songs about dating when I was growing up were so mushy, like, "I love him, I love him, I love him, and where he goes I'll follow, I'll follow, I'll follow." It made me think that you always had to be so excited about the opposite sex and be willing to give up everything for a man.

—PAM, AGE 45

When I was a teenager, I sneaked into an R-rated movie. There was some partial nudity in the movie, and it really turned me on. The actors seemed so free with sex. It was so exciting. It caused me to doubt all the things I had been learning at church.

—PETER, AGE 29

I used to watch this TV show about a group of teenagers who were always teasing and talking about sex. They were all so attractive. They never talked about morality or "waiting." I really felt left out because I hadn't even been kissed yet.

—MARTHA, AGE 24

12. List the various forms of media (e.g., music, magazines, TV, radio, newspapers, movies) that have influenced your feelings and beliefs about sexuality. Next to each medium list what messages about sexuality—both positive and negative—you received.

13. If you have ever looked at pornography in any of its various forms, what messages did it give you about sexuality? Consider the attitudes, personality, and activities of the people portrayed; don't assume that the only messages you picked up were through words.

14. Make a list of the themes about sex and sexual morality that you've internalized from the media and the culture around you. You might be led to believe, for example, that all attractive people are having sex and that it is always fun and exciting. Morality is rarely discussed, and sex seems recreational, just for fun. Sex rarely involves or causes any problems, or

if problems arise, the message is that someone was too careless and got caught.

Peer Group

When I was a young girl, sometimes my friends and I played games like "doctor." We experimented a lot with showing each other our "stuff." We never really touched each other a whole lot, and it seemed just like all of the other play we enjoyed. It didn't seem like a big deal.

—SHANNON, AGE 40

Whenever the guys I knew hung around together, the conversation always turned to sex. Everyone seemed to compare their latest conquests. I never had any of those but used to make some up just to fit in.

—AARON, AGE 26

All the other girls seemed so interested in boys early on. They were so preoccupied with dates and calling boys. I sometimes wondered if there was something wrong with me because boys were not that big a deal to me, even through high school. Some of my friends at school teased me about being "cold."

—AMY, AGE 34

15. When you were growing up, did you ever engage in sexual play with your friends or relatives (cousins, brothers, sisters)? If so, how old were you? What was the nature of the activity? How did it make you feel at the time? How do memories of it make you feel now?

16. As you matured as a boy or a girl, what information did you receive from your friends about sexuality? For example, maybe one of them was the person who first told you about the biology or mechanics of sex. Maybe one of them showed you your first pornography. Did any of your friends help teach you about morality or share a commitment to wait until marriage to have sex? Were you encouraged or teased into being sexual sooner than you wanted?

17. What messages about the roles of males and females did you learn from your friends? Which friends did you emulate in your desire to be "cool" or attractive?

Dating Experience

I remember Virginia, my first love. We went on several dates and really liked each other. She was Catholic, and when her parents found out I was Protestant they forbade her to go out with me anymore. I was crushed and never really much liked Catholics after that.

—MARK, AGE 48

When I was sixteen, I went out with a boy I really liked. One night I got sick at a party, and he was nice enough to take me home right away. On the way, I threw up and was mortified. Even though he asked me out again, I just couldn't go.

—ANN, AGE 27

I was fifteen when I went out on my first date, a double date with my best friend and his date. We went to a drive-in and saw 101 Dalmatians. *It seems so silly and childish now, but we had such a great time.*

—BRAD, AGE 38

I was so excited when a good-looking and popular boy at school became interested in me. He'd meet me between class periods and walk me to my next class. I felt so proud to have a real boyfriend and to be seen with him. After he'd kissed me a few times, however, he seemed to just lose interest. We never talked about it, but next thing I knew he broke up with me. I felt so ashamed. I didn't know what to say to my friends.

—SHEILA, AGE 30

18. As best you can, recall the main dating relationships you have had. What was the nature of your relationships emotionally, sexually, and spiritually? Who was your first love? What kind of disappointments and heartbreaks have you had? Be specific in your journal about your first sexual experi-

ences, however minor they may have seemed, such as your first kiss, first fondling experiences, and so forth.

19. If you had sexual intercourse before you got married, when was that? What has happened to the person or persons with whom you were intimate? Were you ever seriously committed or engaged to someone before you met and married your spouse? What were your feelings for this other person? Are any of them unresolved (e.g., are you still grieving the loss of an earlier love)?

20. If you are divorced, what part did sexuality play in the deterioration of your relationship? Do you think you still carry with you any sexual wounds because of this previous relationship? For example, did your former spouse criticize you sexually? Were you or your former spouse unfaithful? Were there problems with frequency or practice in your sexual relationship? Were you ever forced to do things that you didn't want to do?

Our Shared Dating Experience

I remember going to a football game my senior year in high school and seeing Jenny for the first time. She was one of the new cheerleaders, and I thought she was beautiful, like a goddess. I couldn't get her off my mind for a long time. When we started dating a year later, it was like a miracle.

—STAN, AGE 32

Our first date was a disaster, nothing went right. I didn't really like Jim then, but he kept asking me out, and he was different on later dates when he finally relaxed around me.

—KATHY, AGE 34

When I first met my husband, he was so shy. I noticed, though, that when he smiled he seemed like a really nice guy. When we first went out, what really impressed me were his eyes. He always looked at me as if he really cared.

—DEB, AGE 44

I have to admit, we met at a bar. My husband stood out because he was so tall. I'm embarrassed to say it, but he had a really great body, especially his rear end.

—MARNIE, AGE 25

21. What do you remember about the first time you saw your spouse? What attracted you to him or her in the first place? Think of emotional, spiritual, and physical qualities.

22. When you were dating, what did you do to have fun together? Were you able to "play" together? What did you do that brought you mutual enjoyment? What did you do that made you laugh together? Or were things usually pretty serious?

23. Be as honest as you can about any sexual feelings and experiences you had while you were dating. Were there any tensions between the two of you? How did you deal with them?

24. Make a list of the thoughts and feelings about sexuality and male/female relationships that you experienced with your spouse before you were married. For example:
    • I always seemed to be the one who wanted to be more sexual.
    • I could never seem to get enough.
    • Thank God for my spouse. He/she was the one who always put the brakes on.
    • I didn't really want to have sex, but I went along with it because I thought that's what he/she wanted.
    • I wish that we had waited until we were married to do some of the things that we did.
    • I'm glad that we waited.
    • I always worried that he/she wasn't attracted enough to me physically.
    • He always decided where we were going to go and what we were going to do on dates. He never asked what *I* wanted to do.
    • She was the first girl I'd ever let see me cry. I couldn't believe how safe I felt with her.

- It bugged me that he always expected me to cook him dinner. He much preferred home-cooking to going out to a restaurant. Sometimes I felt like he was looking for a mother.
- He/she always treated me with respect, both in public and in private.

Our Sex Life Together

I was surprised on our honeymoon. The first couple of nights were pretty wild, but then things kind of settled down. It wasn't as passionate as I thought it would be. I think I started being angry at my wife then because she wasn't like all of those videos I had seen. I felt that it really wasn't fair.

—JON, AGE 37

I was really frightened on our wedding night. My friends had told me so many things about what to expect. My husband, though, was really gentle and patient with me. I was so tense that it was hard to enjoy sex at first, but his thoughtfulness over the years has really helped me to relax and experience sex in the fullest sense.

—MARTHA, AGE 35

My husband can't ever seem to get enough. I'm usually available, but lately he has been asking us to do some pretty wild things. He wants me to watch X-rated videos as a way of "spicing up" our sexual relationship. I'm not comfortable with that.

—HANNAH, AGE 31

25. What did you expect your first experience with sexual intercourse with your spouse to be like? What was it actually like? Be as honest as you can.
26. Over the years, what have been the best times sexually with your spouse?
27. Over the years, what have been the worst times sexually?
28. What do you like about your current sexual relationship?
29. What do you dislike?

Other Sexual Experiences

Ever since I was a boy, I seemed to be on fire with sexual thoughts. Maybe lots of these were normal, but I never talked to anyone about them and I thought that I was really terrible. In high school I started using more and more pornography. When I got married, I thought I would stop, but I haven't.

—MARVIN, AGE 40

When I went back to work after our son was born, I never thought that I would have an affair. But the men at work gave me so much attention in ways my husband didn't. It was like things "just happened" on a business trip with Brad last year. Whenever we've gone out of town since then, it has been easier to succumb to temptation since I had already given in.

—SUSAN, AGE 32

I decided to try chat rooms on the Internet, just for fun. I met a man in one of those, and we started e-mailing each other. We were able to tell each other things in relative anonymity that we didn't feel we could tell our spouses. Eventually we exchanged phone numbers and wound up meeting and having sex. Now I can't seem to give up the relationship.

—KATHRYN, AGE 41

30. If you're really brave, make a list of any other sexual experiences you have had. Have you ever masturbated, seen a prostitute, gone to a strip club, had homosexual feelings or experiences, or engaged in some other form of sexual acting out?

31. Do you regularly fantasize? If so, what are your fantasies about?

32. Have you ever or do you now engage in any sexual behaviors in a way that might be considered addictive? If so, describe what this addictive behavior feels and looks like.

33. How have the experiences you wrote about affected your feelings and expectations about sexuality and sexual relationships?

One of the key words that describes sexual addiction is *unmanageable*. Have you ever felt that your sexual feelings or activities are out of control? If so, you may want a professional to evaluate whether or not you have a problem. Never try to diagnose yourself. Call one of the numbers in the resource section and get a phone assessment or a referral to a specialist in your area. You will probably want to talk to a professional counselor or well-trained pastor about how to tell your spouse about these kinds of behaviors. Both of you will need support to deal with this kind of information.

Again you may be wondering, *Why should I go through writing all this down? Why should I relive these past events, feelings, and memories?* My answer to that is twofold. First, these events, feelings, and memories have an effect on you even if it is subconscious. The only way to heal is to be honest about them. You may discover that you need to get professional help. Believe me, if this is the case, you will be giving your children a great gift by getting the help you need. I talk to hundreds of people who discover that their past sexual experiences affect them in so many ways, one of which is how they talk to their spouse and to their children about sex.

Second, being honest about your sexual history is a liberating experience. Carrying around secrets, buried memories, and shame can be a great burden. You may have spent lots of emotional energy wondering what your spouse and other people would think of you if they *really* knew you. I find that in most cases in which people are honest, they draw closer together in the long run.

GROUND RULES FOR A HEALTHY CONVERSATION

Once you have completed your notebooks and are convinced that talking to each other about sex is vital to preparing you to talk with your children about it in a healthy and productive way, then you will be ready to share your feelings, experiences, and beliefs with your spouse. Before you do so, find a trusted friend, counselor, or pastor to consult with about whether or not you are ready, your spouse is ready, and your conversations are prompted by the right reasons. Following are some right and wrong reasons to share information.

Good Reasons	Bad Reasons
• to be more sexually healthy	• to convince my spouse that he or she has a problem
• to become more intimate with my spouse	• to confess my sins so that I can be forgiven right away and get some relief
• to heal past shame	
• to practice talking about sex with someone I love	• to punish my spouse for information he or she has told me
• to practice being honest	
• to understand how to be accountable about sexual faithfulness	• to convince my spouse that he or she needs to be more sexual so that I can control my behavior
• to improve our sexual relationship	
• to prepare both of us to have healthy discussions with our kids about sex	

Right reasons to discuss the things you have written about your past involve building intimacy with your spouse and with your entire family. Wrong reasons are manipulative and self-centered, focused only on personal relief, anger, or blame. Sometimes it's wise to get an outside opinion about our motivation. Discuss with someone you trust what you hope to gain from talking about your history with your spouse. If you get the green light, schedule a meeting with your spouse to talk as a couple. It may take several meetings to discuss everything. If you have written down sensitive information that will come as a surprise to your spouse, you may want to share this information in the presence of a trusted third party who can help you both process your feelings.

You may find that this level of honesty will lead to hurt feelings. Don't be frightened by this. My wife and I have discovered that those periods of time when we have wrestled with the issues closest to our hearts, often with the help of a counselor, have been some of the most intimate and productive hours we have spent. We have benefited, and our children have benefited.

Here are some practical ground rules for a healthy and safe conversation.

1. Be sure to agree on a convenient time and place. Most couples know the time of day when they think or function best and where they feel most comfortable. Make sure to avoid distractions, such as the children being around or the phone ringing. You may not be able to have these discussions at home. My wife and I found that a local restaurant was the best place for us to talk.

2. Agree on a time limit for the conversation. Some people like to talk issues to death. Remember that not all topics have to be "solved." After the time limit is up, reschedule the topic for another time.

3. Don't be afraid of feelings. If they come up, that is good. Many times we get into trouble thinking that we need to "fix" each other. Feelings are not good or bad and don't always need solutions. They are a natural part of life. If my wife is angry with me or sad, it is simply an indication that she cares and is engaged with me. It is not necessary for me to "solve her problem" or talk her out of her feelings.

4. Listen and don't interrupt. Repeat what you've heard, if necessary, so that you can make sure you've understood your spouse correctly.

5. Talk about your own feelings, opinions, and experience. Don't interpret what your spouse thinks, feels, or believes. Never assume anything. Even the best-trained therapists don't make assumptions about what is in people's heads.

6. Avoid blaming. A couple's problems are usually caused by the contributions of both partners. Even if you feel your spouse is clearly in the wrong, always look for your own responsibility.

7. Be affirming. Make an effort to compliment your partner. Maybe it will simply be for saying something honest, even if you don't like what was said.

8. State your needs. Ask for what you would like to have happen based on how you are feeling.

9. Practice. Couples don't automatically know how to have healthy conversations. Even if they think they can, difficult issues (like sexuality) can impair a person's ability to communicate responsibly. I can counsel others in a relatively healthy way, but sometimes when I'm talking to my wife or to one of my children I become like a frightened child. We all need to practice being honest, fair, and mature in our communication. You may want to practice with issues that are not as volatile first and work your way up to those that are more difficult.

10. Get help. When in doubt about how to deal with an issue, find someone who can help you with the conversation. Professional counselors, pastors, or others who have experience with these kinds of issues can help. It is a great sign of strength, not weakness, to ask for help.

Most of all, I would encourage you to begin all conversations with your spouse with words of assurance and affirmation. For example:

"I want you to know that I love you, and I want to be faithful to you emotionally, spiritually, and sexually for the rest of my life. You are the most attractive person in the world to me. Whatever information I share is in no way intended to frighten or hurt you. If it does, please know that I don't intend to do so. I simply want to be honest, to share, and to get to know you better. If I have made mistakes in the past, I will try to correct them in the future. If I need to get help to do so, I will. I surrender my life and our marriage to Christ. I know that God will guide us in this conversation. I hope that you will feel free to be honest

with me. I promise that I will try to listen without blame or condemnation. Nothing you have ever done can cause me to stop loving you."

HEALING TOGETHER

Do you remember Bill and Barbara from the opening story of this chapter? They were having trouble knowing how to talk to their daughter and son about sexuality. Both of them had a sexual past that they had never discussed with each other.

Bill and Barbara heard a sermon one Sunday about parenting. The pastor emphasized that good parents are good models. Bill went home feeling guilty. How could he talk to his son about the evils of pornography when he was so involved with it himself? Barbara, likewise, felt guilty. How could she talk to her daughter about waiting until marriage to be sexual when she hadn't waited herself?

Bill talked to the pastor after the service and scheduled a time to visit with him. He confessed that he struggled with pornography and that he wanted to stop. The pastor told him that a group of men in the church had formed a support group to talk about this very thing. Bill attended this group and found great relief in telling his story for the first time. These men held each other accountable to staying free of pornography. Bill still felt shameful and guilty that he hadn't shared this information with Barbara.

Finally, with the support of the men in his group, Bill worked up the courage to tell Barbara why he was meeting with them. Barbara was hurt in one part of her spirit, but in another part she was also grateful that Bill had been honest enough to tell her. Bill suggested that they go and see their pastor so that he could help them talk through this issue.

Their pastor was a well-trained counselor. He invited both Bill and Barbara to take some time and write the history of their lives and families, including a sexual history. In the safety of their pastor's office, they were finally and slowly able to share this information. Barbara was able to tell Bill, for the first time, about her first sexual expe-

rience before she met him. Likewise, Bill confessed his early sexual experiences. This process took several sessions and at times was quite painful. However, both of them felt incredible relief that they could finally talk openly about their sexual history.

Strangely, Bill found that the more he was able to share both with his men's support group and with Barbara, the less he felt tempted by his lustful thoughts and fantasies. Their pastor advised them to agree to a period of sexual abstinence while they worked on other kinds of intimacy in their relationship. Both of them found that this time of abstinence gave them the freedom to not worry about sex and to concentrate on being honest with each other.

Their pastor also encouraged Bill and Barbara to begin a more energized prayer and Bible study life together. Some of the men in Bill's support group— along with their wives—had been meeting with the pastor. These couples eventually agreed to start meeting together to talk about their healing journeys. It was a wonderful time of fellowship and intimate sharing.

Gradually, Bill and Barbara built a full sexual relationship. Bill found that he was able to be more "present" without fantasizing about other things. Barbara sensed this to be true and knew that her husband was really with her. Even though frequency or technique didn't change all that much, both of them found their sexual relationship much more satisfying.

One day, Bill and Barbara sat down and talked with both of their children. They started the conversation like this: "We want you to know that we haven't always been the best parents that we would like to be. We haven't always talked to you about important things. We're not going to get all of those things talked about tonight. But we do want you to know that we'd like to begin having more honest conversations with you. We want you to be able to talk to us about anything—including sex.

"One of the reasons we haven't felt comfortable doing this before is because we hadn't ever talked to each other about many things, including sex. That may sound strange to you. But even though we've had a sexual relationship, we haven't always been honest with each other. Along the way we may be able to tell you some of the things that we've discovered about our past and about each other. Most of all we want you to know that sex is a wonderful part of marriage that God has given all couples. The fact *that sex is a gift from God is important right now as you date and become interested in the opposite sex. We would like to be your guides and to give you information that is consistent with God's plan for sex. We know we are not perfect; we have made many mistakes. But we love each other and we love you. We hope we can grow together as a family."*

This conversation will lay the groundwork for future discussions. A door is now open to the many teachable moments that will present themselves in the future. At times Bill will need to talk to his son about pornography, and Barbara will talk to her daughter about dating and boys and how to say no. At other times both parents will talk together to one or both of their kids. What a gift these parents will be to their children!

Being able to effectively talk to our children about sex will require that we have a biblically based and mature understanding of what healthy sexuality is. One of the most common mistakes Christians make is to give only a negative perspective on sexuality, to describe only the things we *don't* want our kids to do. We should remember that a normal and natural part of our children's process of growing up is being curious about many things in life, including sex. When parents are negative about sex, normal kids become even more curious about the mysteries of sex and possibly more rebellious in their experimentation.

When we talk to our children about sex, we must strive to teach them a positive perspective about it, one that celebrates sex as a part of the God-ordained relationship between a husband and wife. In the next chapter, we will explore a model of healthy sexuality that will serve as a foundation for the specific conversations you will want to have with your children during each stage of their lives.

CHAPTER TWO

What Is Healthy Sexuality?

Beth and David are the parents of sixteen-year-old Ryan. Since he is an only child, they have always been somewhat overprotective. As Ryan has started dating, their anxieties have hit a new level of intensity. David has talked to Ryan about sex biologically and is convinced that he is well-educated about the mechanics of sex. Ryan has attended church youth group and Sunday school for as long as he can remember. He is familiar with Christian teachings on morality. He knows what not to do.

Lately, Ryan's attention has focused on one particular girl who is also a part of the church youth group. They have started dating and become quite serious with each other. Ryan and his girlfriend have even talked about mutual intentions to abstain from sex. David and Beth still worry about him, however. David remembers back to when he was on fire with physical feelings for Beth before they were married, and he wonders if Ryan feels the same way. He would like to be able to talk to his son about the positive reasons to abstain from premarital sex and what the Bible teaches about sex and intimacy in marriage, but he is at somewhat of a loss as to what to say.

Sometimes it is easier to understand difficult topics by breaking them down into smaller parts. Years ago Ginger Manley, a friend of mine who is a sex therapist in Nashville, defined for me five dimensions of healthy sexuality that I still find helpful in understanding and teaching on this topic (see diagram on next page). The descriptions of these dimensions are my own interpretations. Remember that we are trying to understand healthy sexuality and simply using this division as a way of doing so. With any model we adopt, we must be sure that it can be biblically supported. Therefore, I will also discuss in this chapter what Scripture has to say about healthy sexuality.

Over the years, I have found that the model shown below helps couples to understand the various components of the work they will need to do individually and together to have a healthy sexual relationship. As you begin to understand the model, you will see that healthy sexuality is much more than the physical act of sexual intercourse. The model presents a larger picture of sexuality, one in which the physical act of sexuality is viewed as only one of the expressions of emotional and spiritual intimacy between a husband and wife. Remember, this model is simply a tool. Nothing can fully describe the complete spiritual, emotional, and physical intimacy that married couples can enjoy if their marriage is centered in Christ.

Let's examine each of the dimensions separately.

FIVE DIMENSIONS OF HEALTHY SEXUALITY

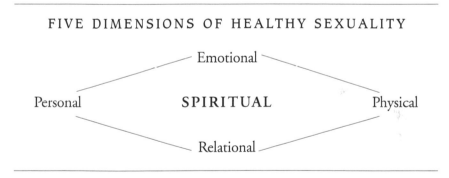

Emotional

Personal   **SPIRITUAL**   Physical

Relational

PHYSICAL DIMENSION

Todd and Erica were a rather normal young Christian couple. Basically, their marriage was going pretty well. However, since her early teen years, Erica had been unhappy with her looks. Her older brothers used to tease her about her development, which was a little slower than some of her friends. This made her rather self-conscious. Todd had tried to affirm her appearance many times, but Erica had a difficult time believing him. More and more she found it harder to be sexual, not really trusting that Todd's sexual drive was out of love for her.

Todd was getting really frustrated. This was not what he thought marriage was going to be like. After waiting to have sex with Erica until after they were married, he now felt cheated and was becoming angrier with his wife all the time. He even found himself being more sexually aggressive with her than he knew was right. He loved his wife and wanted to be more understanding, but as a normal twenty-three-year-old man, he wanted to have sex—and lots of it.

The physical dimension of healthy sexuality assumes that sexual desire is a God-given part of our biology, that there is a natural biological basis to our sexual feelings. In God's design for creation, the stimulus of seeing, smelling, touching, feeling, or hearing the opposite sex will create a physical longing or desire. Physical desire is built into the chemistry of our brains. We need to have it because it is the life force that drives us to reproduce and keep humankind from extinction. Physical desire for each other is a natural part of human sexuality and, therefore, a natural part of a loving marriage.

In the Greek language of the New Testament, three important words are used for our one English word *love: eros, philia,* and *agape.* We'll look at each of these as we survey the five dimensions of healthy sexuality.

First, *eros* describes any physical expression of love between two people. It is the root of our English word *erotic. Eros* is sometimes given a negative connotation and viewed as something to overcome, like sinful lust. The English word *lust* comes directly from a German word that simply means "desire." A person can desire many things, and this is not inherently evil. In English, however, lust has usually come to designate excessive physical desire. Various Hebrew and Greek words have been translated into the word *lust* and generally refer to a combination of physical desire, erotic pleasure, and passion.

The concept of sexual lust is sometimes used in the Bible to describe unbridled and passionate worldly selfishness. For example, Jeremiah describes

Babylon to be like a donkey in heat (Jeremiah 2:24). Paul talks about burning with passion (1 Corinthians 7:9). He says that men dishonor their bodies with the sinful desires of their hearts (Romans 1:24), that we should put to death all evil desires (Colossians 3:5), and that a believer should not lose control of his body in a heathen-like passion of lust (1 Thessalonians 4:4-5). Paul recognizes that young people are prone to evil desires when he tells Timothy to avoid them (2 Timothy 2:22). Peter urges believers to abstain from sinful desires that war against the soul (1 Peter 2:11) and to live according to the will of God (1 Peter 4:2). James says that desire produces sin and sin produces death (James 1:14-15). The point is that the physical desire that is a God-instilled part of our sexuality is a seed that can and does produce much selfishness, sin, and corruption in the world.

However, sexual desire and sexual response are intended by God, in the context of a loving marriage, for procreation and pleasure. We should never be afraid or ashamed of natural physical attraction and desire. We need to teach our children this. We must be careful not to convey the idea that physical attraction and desire are evil. At the same time, we must explain that our natural brain chemistry is not intended to drive us like mere animals. Biblically, going back to the Garden of Eden, it is the work of the devil that takes human desire and turns it into a selfish demand for immediate gratification. God also, therefore, has created us with a spirit and has given us a set of instructions that can help us to override our biological chemistry, a matter that requires discipline and practice. We need to teach our children that while it is normal to have sexual desire, people must learn to focus their desire on one person, a husband or a wife, and put that person's needs first. This is a spiritual process.

The apostle Paul explained why what we do with our bodies is so important:

> Do you not know that your bodies are members of Christ himself? Shall I then take the members of Christ and unite them with a prostitute? Never! Do you not know that he who unites himself

> with a prostitute is one with her in body? For it is said, "The two will become one flesh." But he who unites himself with the Lord is one with him in spirit.
>
> Flee from sexual immorality. All other sins a man commits are outside his body, but he who sins sexually sins against his own body. Do you not know that your body is a temple of the Holy Spirit, who is in you, whom you have received from God? You are not your own; you were bought at a price. Therefore honor God with your body. (1 Corinthians 6:15-20)

Any understanding of sexuality should begin here.

Temples are sacred places. They are sanctuaries. Another definition for sanctuary is "safe place." We should always attempt to keep our bodies sacred and safe places. As parents, our job is to help our children learn how to do this. As responsible parents, we teach our children about private parts of their body that they should be very careful to protect. We educate them about the dangers of sexual abuse. We warn them about improper situations and advances. We can describe the improper use of power that some may use physically, emotionally, or spiritually to gain sexual access to them. We should also teach them that their bodies are gifts from God and temples they will each want to share with only one other person. Finally, sanctuaries should be lovingly maintained. Our bodies, as temples, should be properly cared for. This is a matter of physical care such as preventive medicine, healthy diet and habits, rest, and exercise.

Paul also stressed the importance of honoring the body (temple) of one's spouse:

> The husband should fulfill his marital duty to his wife, and likewise the wife to her husband. The wife's body does not belong to her alone but also to her husband. In the same way, the husband's body does not belong to him alone but also to his wife. (1 Corinthians 7:3-4)

This is one of the passages that many of us can abuse, particularly men. We can use it to demand sex. What I think Paul was really talking about, however, is that we should honor and respect our partner's body. He recognized that sexual feeling is normal and that most people will marry. He was not saying, however, that we should be consumed by sexual demands in marriage. Our partner's body is also a temple of the Holy Spirit, and we should honor it just as we would any sacred place. We should strive to make sexual expression "safe" for our partners. This may mean that we place the safety and comfort of our partner above our own selfish desire.

In Ephesians 5, *before* Paul talked about submission of wives and husbands to one another, he said this:

> And live a life of love, just as Christ loved us and gave himself up
> for us as a fragrant offering and sacrifice to God.... Among you
> there must not be even a hint of sexual immorality, or of any kind
> of impurity, or of greed, because these are improper for God's
> holy people. (verses 2-3)

Paul's vision of love involves sacrifice: Just as Christ died for us, we must sometimes kill our selfish desires in honor of our spouse. It is only through love, not by demands or control, that healthy physical sexuality flourishes.

Finally, Paul offered us a balanced perspective about our bodies:

> But we have this treasure in jars of clay to show that this all-
> surpassing power is from God and not from us. We are hard
> pressed on every side, but not crushed; perplexed, but not in
> despair; persecuted, but not abandoned; struck down, but not
> destroyed. We always carry around in our body the death of
> Jesus, so that the life of Jesus may also be revealed in our body.
> (2 Corinthians 4:7-10)

Even temples are perishable. They are "earthen vessels." We should never honor our bodies more than we do the spirit inside. Go to the nearest health club, and you will find people honoring their bodies as temples, but many of them are forgetting that there is a spirit inside. We should always help our children to know that whatever their appearance, they are precious in the sight of God and that their spirit is the most vital component in their overall health.

EMOTIONAL DIMENSION

Paul and Cathy had a great sexual relationship, or so they thought. They had read all the manuals and were generally fun-loving and creative. They thought they were the perfect couple since they had sex frequently, usually enjoyed it, and were excited by it. They also believed that as long as the sex was good, their marriage must be good, so they generally ignored all advice and teaching about having more communication and spirituality in their relationship. They didn't think anything of the fact that they seemed to be drifting into questionable kinds of sexual activity. Paul would occasionally bring home a video so they could get new ideas. This all seemed harmless.

As the months and years went by, however, even the newest activities seemed boring. Sex wasn't as much fun anymore. The only fantasy that seemed to bring any sense of excitement—to Paul, at least—was the thought of a new partner.

Paul and Cathy were on a very slippery slope, with one or both of them sliding toward an affair. What they didn't realize is that, while their physical sexual activity was varied and creative, the two of them shared little emotional or spiritual communication.

Obviously, healthy sexuality is more than just bodies uniting together; it is also a matter of ever-deepening intimacy. It demands that we are honest with our husband or wife and that we seek to be "present" with them.

In Genesis 2:24, the foundation of marriage is described: "For this reason a man will leave his father and mother and be united to his wife, and they will become one flesh." To me this is more than just an image of sexual intercourse. It means that the husband and wife become one in mind and spirit. This oneness requires being totally "known" to each other. In fact, in some translations of the Bible, the word *know* is synonymous with sexual intercourse.

As I pointed out in the first chapter, this kind of intimacy is not easy for many couples to attain and practice. Really knowing each other requires that we be honest about what we truly think and feel, and that demands vulnerability. The word *vulnerable* comes from the Latin word *vulnus,* which means "wound." To let another person really know us involves taking the risk that we might be wounded by their reaction. Many people go to elaborate lengths to avoid taking that risk. One of the keys to the emotional dimension, then, is how well we can deal with our fear of really being known.

How effectively are you, as parents, modeling intimacy for your children? Do they see you talking in caring and loving ways to each other, or do they see you avoiding issues and being distant? Do you model unhealthy behaviors, even addictions, that teach them about avoiding or medicating their feelings? If you are to be successful at teaching your kids to value healthy intimacy in relationships, including the relationship with their future spouses, then you'll need to do your best to model it for them, first with your spouse and then with your kids.

Here is a checklist of ways to demonstrate intimacy as you interact.

1. Talk *with* your kids, not *at* them. Be a good listener. (This rule applies to interactions with your spouse as well!)
2. Don't demand that your kids answer your questions. Give them the freedom to talk when they feel safe to do so.
3. Admit to your kids when you have been wrong. Don't be afraid that they will use this admission against you later. Don't model blaming behavior in front of them. Accept responsibility. Model how to make changes and/or restitution for mistakes you have made. Children will respect a person who knows how to admit failure and is willing to make changes. They don't need perfect parents.

4. Talk with your kids about your feelings. Describe to them times when you have been angry, lonely, frightened, or sad. Don't expect them to "fix" your feelings. It is even appropriate to shed tears in front of children as long as they don't feel the responsibility to solve your problems.

5. Allow your children to be angry with you. Teach them how to do this in acceptable ways that are not damaging to you or others. Model healthy expressions of anger in ways that are neither physically violent nor emotionally dramatic.

6. When your children are sad, lonely, or frightened, don't try to talk them out of it or solve their problems for them. Listen, listen, listen!

7. Demonstrate problem-solving skills to your kids. Help them define the true nature of problems, show them alternative solutions, and teach them a process for reaching a decision. Allow them to fail at their decisions as long as that failure won't bring permanent consequences.

As you teach your children to be honest by modeling with your spouse and with them how to risk sharing their feelings with others, they will learn about the kind of emotional intimacy that is crucial to healthy adult sexuality.

RELATIONAL DIMENSION

Richard and Andrea met at a bar during their college years. They are both physically attractive, and the sexual energy between the two of them was palpable from the start. They enjoyed flirting at the bar, and then they went to Andrea's apartment and became sexual. The next few weeks were a torrid sexual adventure—wild, passionate, and creative. It felt like love, they were so sexually compatible. Everything was so great, they decided to get married!

Richard and Andrea finished college and began thinking about having children. Andrea soon got pregnant. This changed things sexually between them. Richard grew restless, and Andrea resented that he didn't understand. Things degenerated as more kids came along. Richard and Andrea went through a periodic cycle in which they would get more and more resentful of each other, have a major blowup, and then make up, which also led to great sex.

During the ninth year of their marriage, they were discipled by another couple and became Christians. They hoped that accepting Christ would cure all of their problems. What they didn't realize is how much of a sexual foundation their marriage had been built on. They had never really talked to each other. They had no concept of friendship or intimacy.

Fortunately, other couples in their church talked to them about and modeled friendship to them. As they studied Scripture about friendship love (philia), *they began to try to practice biblical principles with each other. Part of this process of discovery was a commitment to go on a sexual fast (abstinence) together. In order to become friends, they had to temporarily take sex out of the equation and begin to rebuild their relationship from the ground up. This fast lasted about three months.*

The first time they made love after this, they were amazed that it was a whole different experience. For one thing, even in the midst of sex, they looked each other in the eyes for the first time and felt that they were beginning to really know each other. Their lovemaking was not as wildly exciting, but it was gentler, kinder, and more patient. They both seemed more interested in satisfying each other. It was so totally different and deeper than anything they had ever done. Afterward, they both wept with joy.

On their tenth anniversary, they stood before their pastor, friends from the church, and their children and renewed their vows.

There are several aspects of a healthy marital relationship; physical sex and emotional intimacy are only two. The second Greek word for love, *philia,* describes another aspect of a well-rounded relationship: friendship in the form of brotherhood or sisterhood. A husband and wife should be friends, a brother and sister in Christ who become one flesh. For example, in 1 Peter 3, Peter gave some rather clear advice to husbands and wives. In this context, he wrote in verse 8, "Finally, all of you, live in harmony with one another; be sympathetic, love as brothers, be compassionate and humble." If you were to do a word search of the Bible for the words *brother* or *sister,* you would find that most commentaries refer you to other words like *communion, patience, compassion, kindness,* and *love (philia).*

Perhaps the clearest description of this kind of love was given to us by Paul in 1 Corinthians 13 when he said, "Love is patient, love is kind. It does not envy, it does not boast, it is not proud. It is not rude, it is not self-seeking, it is not easily angered, it keeps no record of wrongs. Love does not delight in evil but rejoices with the truth. It always protects, always trusts, always hopes, always perseveres. Love never fails" (verse 4-8).

In Galatians 5:22-23, Paul described the "fruit of the Spirit": love, joy, peace, patience, kindness, goodness, faithfulness, gentleness, and self-control. How can I improve on the teachings of Paul? He is teaching us how we should love each other as brothers and sisters in Christ. Certainly, all of these qualities are things that husbands and wives should strive for with each other. This is *philia* love. This kind of love is one of the antidotes to the greed of selfish lust.

What does it mean then to be friends? Following are several components of healthy friendship given to us by Paul. Friends are:
- patient with each other, self-controlled, peaceful, and persevering;
- kind to each other and not rude;
- not proud or boastful, always looking to take personal responsibility;
- gracious and forgiving, keeping no record of past wrongs or delighting in current failures;
- not jealous or envious of each other;
- trusting of each other;
- committed to being truthful with each other;
- slow to anger and quick to resolve conflict;
- hopeful and steadfast; and
- joyous.

To teach your children about healthy marriage, let me suggest some practical things you can do as a couple to model *philia* love.

Affirm each other in their presence. Be cheerleaders for each other and support each other as best friends.

Don't be afraid to fight in front of them. The word *fight* can be misleading. Parents who know how to express anger to each other in healthy ways aren't really fighting. When they are angry, they say so in nonblaming and nondestructive ways. They don't yell, scream, blame, hit, or pout. A healthy fight is civil and gets resolved relatively quickly.

My wife and I didn't used to handle anger very well. We would store it up for months, and then it would explode in a major way. We never got physically violent with each other, but it could sure be dramatic. We had read Christian authors who advised that a couple should never let the sun set on their anger, but our fights would usually end up with me trying to talk an issue to death and Deb feeling like she needed to get away. No one had ever really shown us how to share our anger or resentment in constructive ways. Of course, one of the things that we were angry about was sex. I wanted more and was always pushy. Our inability to talk in healthy ways about sex, or any other subject, would leave us in very bad places, and our kids witnessed this. Gradually, however, we have learned to tell each other about our anger and hurts, and we know that those feelings don't mean that either one of us wants a divorce.

You won't always have your fights in front of the kids, and you will never want to alarm them. But by modeling healthy conflict resolution, you will be sending a powerful message that friends can resolve even the most difficult problems.

Play together. Show your kids how much fun you have together. Friends enjoy each other's company and bring joy to each other's lives.

Many couples talk to me about not having a playful or spontaneous sexual relationship. Their problem is often that they don't know how to play, period. Many adults forget how to play. Perhaps they were expected to become grown-up too early in their lives. My wife once gave me a picture of herself when she was three. The back of the picture said, "Would you like to come out and play?" I didn't quite know what she meant, but it did sound challenging. So I thought about tennis or golf or something that I could compete at. But that is not really play. Play is doing silly things that don't matter at all. So we rolled down a hill together, swung on swings, blew bubbles, and had a pillow fight. It is amazing what playfulness can do for a sexual relationship.

Parents who don't know how to play usually don't play with their children either. Those of you who have forgotten how to play, or who never really knew how in the first place, will need to practice. Your children can be your built-in consultants. Modeling joy to them may mean getting down on the floor, even together as a couple, and playing at their level. Include them in your couple playtime. You need to show them that Mom and Dad have joy together, that they enjoy being with each other, and that they laugh together.

Be affectionate with each other. Close friends are physically affectionate with each other in healthy ways, ways that don't involve sexual touch or intercourse. I work with many men and women who have come to depend on sexual activity as the only way they have their need for touch met. This can wreak havoc with marriages. For example, a person who is overly sexually aggressive with his or her spouse may simply need to be held or touched. Sometimes problems with addiction to masturbation, pornography, prostitution, or other forms of sexual sin have their roots in a lack of healthy nonsexual touch. Sexual sin can be a desperate attempt to be touched and nurtured.

Model healthy sexuality to your kids by touching each other in nonsexual ways. Hugging, handholding, an arm around the shoulder, and even a kiss on the cheek can show your children that you know how to affirm one another in intimate but nonsexual ways. And don't forget to affirm your kids in these ways as well. Our children's healthy development and the health of their sexual relationship in marriage can depend on being touched in nonsexual ways as they are growing up.

Have a spiritual life together. Pray together. Study Scripture together and let your kids see that. Brothers and sisters in Christ nurture each other's spiritual lives and worship God together.

Complement each other. Friends know each other's strengths and weaknesses and mutually complement each other. A husband and wife, likewise, know each other and how they work together best. This partnership involves making practical decisions about how they earn and manage money, wash clothes, cook meals, clean and maintain a home, and care for their children. Show your kids how friends cooperate in a productive way.

Have other friends besides your spouse. A common problem in many marriages is that spouses become too dependent on each other. I have worked with many couples who simply don't have any intimate friends outside of their marriage. They may have lots of social acquaintances, but they don't have real fellowship. Men need to have male friends, other men they can talk to about their problems. Likewise, women need to have fellowship with other women. Couples need to have other couples that they form a community with. When a couple doesn't have these things, the strain on their marriage can be profound.

Having friendships with other believers also provides husbands and wives with accountability. Some of us think of accountability only as having our hands slapped if we don't do something we have agreed to do. To me, accountability has more to do with having a group of friends who will help us to follow through with goals and strategies we have for ourselves. One of my goals, for example, is to stay sexually faithful to my wife. I need to be held accountable to that goal. That means I have a fellowship of men who help me remain faithful and true. One of the basic principles I teach couples is that fellowship equals freedom from lust. If being lonely and isolated or feeling unloved and untouched leads to sexual sin, then having a community of friends is one of the antidotes.

When we teach our children that they are part of not only a biological family, but of a larger community of believers, we will be establishing them on firm footing. As you will see in later chapters, it is vital that young people know how to establish a healthy community of friends for themselves. If they can't, they are more vulnerable to peer pressure that may lure them into sinful behavior of all kinds in order to be accepted. Imagine the pressure of thinking that being sexual is the ultimate way to be loved. Parents who want to teach their children to wait for sex must show them that *philia* love is valuable and fulfilling.

It has been said that true love consists not of two people gazing at each other, but of two people looking together in the same direction. God calls couples beyond just being friends with each other to fellowship with and ministry to others. Let your kids see you interacting with and caring about the church and community beyond your own family so they will learn the value of community.

It is clear to me from working with hundreds of couples that many treat other people better than they treat their spouses. No marriage can be built on sex alone or on the shared responsibility of raising a family. Couples who don't practice *philia* love with each other will eventually have sexual problems. Couples who do love each other as friends will be able to develop a sex life that is much deeper than anything we see in the movies.

PERSONAL DIMENSION

Sharon was sexually molested by her stepfather between the ages of eleven and thirteen. Her mother knew something was going on, but Sharon never told her directly, and her mom never pursued it. When Sharon asked her mom to talk to her husband about something comparatively "minor" (walking in on her while she was bathing), her mom told her she shouldn't be so modest and that "families" weren't embarrassed about such things.

By the time Sharon was a teenager, she hated men, especially her stepdad. She wanted to be part of the social scene at school, but when she went out with boys she always felt uncomfortable, even hostile. After a few dates, most boys gave up and moved on. Sharon felt their rejection, yet she was always strangely relieved.

Mike seemed different. They met as seniors in high school, and she found him easy to talk to. He didn't pressure her sexually, and he genuinely seemed to care about her feelings and to want to get to know her mind. They became best friends and married two years later.

Their sexual problems started almost immediately. No matter how gentle and patient Mike was—and he was indeed a wonderful, godly man—Sharon could not respond to him sexually. The minute sexual activity would begin, she would shut down emotionally and feel like she was floating far from her body, watching their lovemaking from afar. She knew Mike was devastated by her inability to love him as a wife should, but she felt helpless to change.

Sharon and Mike's relationship is an example of the emotional and sexual effects of an unhealed wound. Those, like Sharon, who have been sexually abused will often shut down totally as a way of trying to control the pain of the past. Others who have been hurt may turn around as adults and become the sexual aggressors. Victims of sexual abuse believe that as long as they are in control, either by being active and aggressive or by being sexually shut down, everything will be safe.

Any form of deep personal wounding will affect a couple's sexual relationship. Some wounds have come through invasion—emotional, physical, sexual, or spiritual. Sharon clearly had experienced invasion from her stepfather. Other wounds are the result of being abandoned emotionally, physically, or spiritually. This is a hard wound to describe. How does one know what he has missed if he never had it? How do you describe zero? Such a wound feels like a deep void and loneliness in a person's soul. Sharon had a huge void related to both her mother's abdication of responsibility to keep Sharon safe and her mother's complete emotional abandonment.

Many other forms of wounds can create problems with sexual desire, preference, or orientation. Having a healthy sexual relationship in marriage requires that these wounds be addressed and healed. We must teach our children how to be safe and how to heal any wounds in their human spirit.

SPIRITUAL DIMENSION

Mary's husband had been emotionally and physically abusive to her for years, and he became especially forceful when it came to sex.

When they both became Christians, Mary prayed that her husband would find a kinder and gentler way. One night when she had the flu, she told her husband that she just couldn't be sexual. The next morning he taped up pieces of paper all over the house in places that she would be sure to see. On every piece of paper were just three words: 1 Corinthians 7.

Mary's husband is not the first Christian man to misunderstand and misuse biblical truth like the admonition in 1 Corinthians that tells us to fulfill our "marital duties" in the bedroom and "not deprive each other except by mutual consent." Spouses have quoted Scripture verses out of context for centuries in order to sexually manipulate each other. Obviously, this is not what God intended. So what did God really want when he created males and females to become "one flesh" in marriage?

Even Paul admits that the idea of "one flesh" is "a profound mystery." However, he reveals that it ultimately reflects the relationship between Christ and the church (Ephesians 5:32). Christ didn't come to earth just to say, "Here are my demands and you are to be obedient." Christ came to die for his bride, the church. Following his example in the marital relationship then, means sacrificing for and serving one another. If we think of healthy marital sexuality in these terms, we are really talking about being totally unselfish as we meet each other's needs. Sex should not be the highest priority. Rather, we are to strive to be Christlike with each other, to love each other as we love ourselves (Galatians 5:14).

The spiritual dimension of healthy sexuality prescribes that we reach beyond physical love, *eros,* and friendship, *philia,* to true spiritual love, *agape. Agape* is the word used by the apostle John in 1 John 4:8: "God is love." Nurturing the one-flesh spiritual nature of marriage requires the spiritual discipline of working to keep God in the center of the relationship. Do we know how to pray together, study Scripture together, and talk together about God? For some of us, these activities aren't easy. Personally, I can pray, preach, or talk with thousands of people, but ask me to pray with my wife and I might panic. Prayer and other forms of deeply spiritual communication are difficult and frightening for most of us because they represent the highest form of intimacy.

If the only connection a couple has is a physical or genital one, the relationship is doomed to failure. But when a couple achieves spiritual intimacy, physical intimacy becomes infused with it. The act of genital sexuality can be a spiritual connection. Attaining this spiritual connection requires that both husband and wife are committed to Christ and that together they submit their marriage to Christ. Children who are raised in homes where this is the case should be able to discern the spiritual love their parents have for each other. This is the most profound of models and will provide children with a vision of what they can have in their own marriages someday.

In chapters 4–8, I will return to this five-pronged model of healthy sexuality—physical, emotional, relational, personal, and spiritual—and apply it to each stage of a child's life. But first, let's explore some basic communication principles you'll need to embrace in order to have a lifetime of effective conversations with your kids.

CHAPTER THREE

Principles for Healthy Conversation

Gary and Kathy had three children ages three, six, and eleven. All of them were becoming curious about sex at different developmental levels. Gary and Kathy had tried to respond to the occasional sexual questions or situations that occurred, but neither had ever initiated a conversation with their children about sex.

One day Kathy took all three of the children to the local shopping mall. Three-year-old Molly saw a pregnant woman and asked her mom why she was "so fat." At the same mall, six-year-old Matthew asked why there were so many pictures of women in their underwear. In the video store, Kathy found eleven-year-old Scott studying the covers of soft-core pornographic movies.

Kathy wished that Gary was with them. To Molly, she simply said that she would someday understand. To Matthew, she just sighed, "I really don't know. It's embarrassing, isn't it?" She was much harder on Scott, "Stop looking at that! You know it's evil."

Later that night when Kathy told her husband about the day's events, Gary wanted to talk to his children. He was really angry with Scott about the pornography. He also felt guilty because he still struggled with pornography himself. He felt really frightened and couldn't understand why. The next day, he remembered that, when he was twelve, his dad had once beaten him with a belt for looking at pornography.

Kathy also had mixed feelings. Mainly she was angry about Scott because she knew that her own husband struggled with pornography. Not only was she embarrassed by Matthew's question about underwear, she was pained by the memories it prompted of a time Gary brought home some skimpy items from Victoria's Secret and asked her to dress for him in the same kind of lingerie that the women in the catalog wore. She was also vaguely sad and lonely. She simply couldn't remember how her own mother had handled sexual questions with her. She was not even sure how to respond to Molly's natural curiosity about pregnancy.

Many parents can relate to Kathy and Gary's discomfort and uncertainty when it comes to talking with their kids about even the basics of human sexuality. Most of us want to teach our children well and feel comfortable doing so; but even when we've done the hard work of talking to each other and have a good understanding of healthy sexuality, we can still feel at a loss as to how to have a productive conversation. Following is a discussion of some of the principles of healthy conversation that I've found are particularly useful for parents. Let's look at each one in light of the challenges Kathy and Gary's kids presented to them during a typical family outing to the mall.

Listen, Especially for the Hidden Questions

Parents often tell me that their children never ask sexual questions. In various workshops, participants have said that whenever, as adults, they have approached their parents about why they never talked about sexuality, the parents have responded, "You never asked." The main problem here is that most children don't know how to ask the right questions. In the story above, for example, was eleven-year-old Scott supposed to say, "Dad, I was wondering if you could tell me something about the testosterone that seems to be pulsating through my body." Was the three-year-old supposed to say, "Mom, could you explain pregnancy and reproduction to me?" Was the six-year-old expected to ask, "Why do advertisers use sex appeal so often?"

Since we parents don't hear specific, articulate questions, we often assume that we must do all the talking. So we do our duty by giving our children basic information, and then we assume that since they don't ask questions directly, they have all the information they need. Like Kathy and Gary, however, we often fail to listen between the lines and to respond to what might be going on inside our children's heads.

Here is a list of questions and statements that might be appropriate conversation-starters with your child:

- How do you feel when you see that?
- What do you think that means?
- Have others been talking to you about these things?
- That's a really good question.
- That reminds me of a time when I was your age.
- That takes me back to some real confusion I had.
- That must be really hard to understand.

You probably know that when you feel someone else is really listening to you, it is much easier to talk. Later chapters in this book will help you to understand your children's frame of reference and respond to them accordingly. One of the best questions to ask yourself is, "When I was (my child's age) what did I need? What would have been helpful for me to hear? What information did I need? What would have calmed my fears?"

Emphasize the Positives

Like the other principles I'm sharing here, this is a good strategy for all parenting and all human relationships for that matter. I am continually amazed at how many people are starved for affirmation. Think of people in your life who have been sources of inspiration to you. My guess is that they were affirming. I don't intend to imply that there are never times to deliver a tough message or instruct with discipline. However, beginning with something positive is a very good way to help a person feel safe enough to hear whatever you have to say.

When your child does something you like, tell her so. Even when you want to correct a mistake or problem behavior, it is not a bad idea to begin with a positive statement. Sometimes when you are angry or embarrassed by a behavior, finding a positive approach will be harder. Take time out for yourself and respond later.

In Kathy's situation, for example, an affirming response could have started with a simple statement. When Matthew commented on all the pictures of people clothed in underwear, she might have said, "You're really observant. It does seem to be true that there are." When Molly pointed out the "fat" woman, Kathy could have said, "It's interesting to see so many different kinds of people, isn't it? I'd like to explain a little more to you about why that woman has a big tummy. After Daddy gets home tonight, we'll talk about it together." Gary might have affirmed Scott by saying, "I know what it's like to be attracted to those kind of videos. I was like that when I was your age. It's pretty normal." Any further explanation or discipline may proceed after a child believes that he or she isn't "bad" for being curious or asking questions.

Never Talk About Something You Are Trying to Teach When You're Angry

So many wounds can be inflicted in anger. Remember times in your own life when someone was trying to teach you something (it may even have been the right thing), but you simply didn't hear it because that person was angry. All you felt was fear. So it is with your children.

Gary could have frightened and injured Scott just as his own father had wounded him when he was young. Scott doesn't need to be shamed for his curious behavior, which is very normal for his age. But Gary will need to have many discussions with Scott about the dangers of pornography and how to make healthy spiritual decisions about sexual situations. Being angry and threatening about Scott's curiosity might have the opposite effect Gary intends. In Scott's mind it may make him wonder, "Why did Dad get so angry about that?" He may think, "That wasn't a big deal. Dad's kind of crazy." Scott may also be angered by his father's words and think defiantly,

"I'll show him. I'm going to look at that stuff whenever I want to." The outcome for Scott will probably be much more positive if he feels loved and affirmed in the process of being instructed and disciplined by his dad.

Eleven-year-old Ben was having a hard time going to sleep. He had an active mind but did not yet have the maturity to know how to turn it off. So he would stay up all night and watch TV or play one of his computer games. His parents were simply fried. They tried to set boundaries. Without going into detail, they pointed out how many dangerous things were on TV and the Internet at night. They told Ben to go to bed and made sure he went there. But eventually they had to sleep. They felt they had no privacy or downtime of their own.

When Ben finally went to bed, he would lie there and become more and more anxious. "Why can't I go to sleep?" Ben didn't know what to do. He became like a three-year-old having a temper tantrum. Many nights he would pound his fist against the wall. He was so angry that he couldn't get to sleep. This in turn made his parents even more angry. They sometimes thought it was just a game Ben played to manipulate them into letting him stay up and watch or do the wrong things. This behavior went on for months.

One night Ben's dad was standing in his son's bedroom, on the verge of a violent rage, when a voice inside stopped him. A memory flashed into his head of all those lonely nights when he couldn't go to sleep when he was a kid. He thought, "What did I need back then?" He went over to his son's bed and grabbed him in a hug so tight that Ben couldn't get away. He struggled, but his dad wouldn't let him go. He just kept whispering in his son's ear, "I love you." After thirty seconds Ben began to melt, and several minutes later he was asleep.

What Ben needed was touch and safety. He needed to be loved. A lot of crazy behavior gets started late at night when people are tired, lonely, frightened, and bored.

Always remember that, in any given situation, what is much more important than your words is your attitude. Your words may be exactly correct theologically, psychologically, and in every other way, but if you say them in anger or frustration, that is what your child will remember.

Don't Put Off an Answer Forever

Three-year-olds, like Molly, have a different perception of time than adults do. She certainly doesn't know what her mother's response about "someday understanding" means. She is curious and wants her question answered *now*.

When parents are caught off guard or are embarrassed by a question or situation, the temptation is to say, "We'll talk about that later…" and then never get around to "later." It is not a bad strategy to take time to think about an answer. Deferring an immediate response will also allow a couple time to confer about an appropriate answer and then talk to their child together. Sometimes it is not advisable to put off an impatient child, however. He or she might be tempted to think, "That must be a stupid question I asked or else Mom or Dad would have answered it," or "Why does Mom or Dad seem so impatient with me? Why did that question make them so angry (or embarrassed)?"

Sometimes when you don't answer sexual questions directly, your response only serves to increase a child's curiosity and the sense of danger and mystery surrounding sex. Therefore, be direct when asked simple questions. Answer them immediately. Molly's question, on the other hand, is important and demands a thoughtful answer that addresses where babies come from. For important questions about sexuality, you may want to delay the full explanation while assuring your child that you are glad she asked and that you will answer her question as soon as you've had some time to think about it.

Note from Molly's question how early we may need to think about giving a child information. Molly is not an unusual child. She will observe other pregnant women and will have the same question until she gets some kind of answer.

Gary and Kathy sat down with Molly and said, "We want to explain about why that lady today seemed so fat. She really wasn't fat. You see, she has a baby inside of her. Before they are born, babies grow inside their mothers, in a special place called a uterus, until they are ready to come out. This is the way God planned for babies to start." Gary and Kathy had a picture of Kathy when she was pregnant with Molly. "Molly, this is Mom when you were inside of her. See, she had a big tummy too."

Molly may have many other questions at this point, such as "How did I get in Mom's tummy?" Her parents will need to be ready with a very basic explanation of where babies come from, even at this age. We will talk about these things in chapter 4.

Don't Force Your Kids to Talk

Let's assume that Gary didn't handle the situation well with Scott. He might have said, "That wasn't the first time you've looked at this stuff, was it? How long have you been doing this? Are the other boys doing this too? You don't have any magazines or videos in your room, do you? What were you thinking about? Tell me how that stuff makes you feel."

Scott is going to feel invaded. He won't want to answer these questions and will feel embarrassed and ashamed. He may want to protect friends. This approach is no way to encourage trust or provide an opportunity for Scott to share with his dad what's going on with him.

As they grow up, kids are in the process of establishing their own identities. They will need to find a greater and greater sense of independence and to feel increasingly responsible for their own actions. Sometimes, having secrets is a part of feeling independent. When we rob our children of their ability to have their own lives, we may propel them into more rebellious attitudes than those they already have. We will need to be careful. We don't want to allow sinful or destructive behavior, but at times we need to back off and trust that we will have many other opportunities to offer our instruction and example.

Tell Stories

Stories appeal to the child in all of us. They reveal truth in ways that we can understand. Jesus was a master storyteller. Even though you may not be able to remember chapter and verse, you may be able to remember some of the parables Jesus told. It has always been interesting to me that Jesus never wrote anything down. He never got involved in long theological debates with the educated people around him. They continually tried to test him with difficult questions. In response he usually told stories or created word pictures to help his listeners get to the heart of the issue at hand.

Culture often teaches us about sexuality through stories. Consider the sexual messages we pick up through current news stories, movies, TV shows, books, and other media. Many of the stories that popular culture has to tell are far off the mark, to say the least, from what we want our children to learn about healthy sexuality. One of the best ways to combat the onslaught of the stories the media tells is to tell different stories to our children.

I suggest starting with Bible stories. I had a professor in seminary who took us through the entire Old Testament in one semester simply by telling us the stories it records. Taught in that context, the Bible came alive for me with the story of God's relationship with his people. This professor was a master storyteller. I don't remember one thing he said about the Hebrew derivation of words or the archaeology of certain places, such as where Moses crossed the Red Sea. I do remember the stories. There was a spiritual presence about that teacher, an awe and wonder about God's design that infused his storytelling. Do you have sense of wonder? Part of your preparation as parents may be to study God's story together.

My own father never talked much to me about sex, but he, too, was a great storyteller. At night when I went to bed, instead of telling me fairy tales he would make the Bible come alive by telling me stories. I think back on that today and know that much of my early love of the Bible came from my father's own love of stories.

The Bible, mainly the Old Testament, is full of stories about sex. Think about the fact, for example, that the first man of God's new covenant people, Abraham, committed incest (Genesis 20:12). God's strongest man, Samson, went to see a prostitute (Judges 16:1) and had an unhealthy relationship. God's greatest king, David, was a voyeur and committed murder to cover up an affair (2 Samuel 11). God's wisest man, Solomon, "loved many…women" (1 Kings 11:1). In the New Testament, one of the great lessons about grace is the story of how Jesus dealt with an adulterous woman (John 8:1-11).

Gary and Kathy could have drawn on the story of Elizabeth, the mother of John, and Mary, the mother of Christ, to talk to their daughter about pregnancy. I love the part about John leaping in Elizabeth's womb when the pregnant Mary greets her (Luke 1:41). You will probably not want to get into a conversation with a three-year-old about the Virgin Birth, but it is a fun story about how babies live first in their mother's wombs.

In addition to the Bible, find stories from modern culture and your own life experience that depict people of faith and healthy sexual morality. I realize that you may need to dig for these. We don't sell many products today by saying, "If you wear this or do this, you will stay sexually faithful." The evening news usually doesn't start with, "Our top story tonight is about a couple who just celebrated their fiftieth wedding anniversary," or "Tonight we bring you details of how our president avoided sexual sin in the Oval Office." Nevertheless, people of faith are out there. Make it your business to be resourceful and creative. Your kids need to hear stories about healthy and godly sexuality.

Be Willing to Tell Your Own Story

One of the most common mistakes that many parents make is thinking that if they tell their children about their own struggles or mistakes, their confession will come back to haunt them, or their children will not respect them. My experience is that nothing is further from the truth. Ask yourself the question, "If my parents had shared their own journey with me, how would I have felt?" Remember that one of the main thoughts of a lonely person is, "I'm the only one having this thought or experience." What a relief it can be to know that he or she is not the only one! This is particularly true with sexual thoughts. How often has someone thought that she is the biggest sexual sinner or pervert in the world because of a rather common thought that slipped into her mind? If a person doesn't know that something is normal, how tempting it is to believe that he is a terrible person.

I believe that it is a moral imperative for parents to tell their children some of their own stories. There is good and bad timing for this, of course. Your story should be shared at age-appropriate times. You wouldn't share an adolescent experience with a three-year-old or an adult experience with an adolescent. You would never want to share your story if you are just looking for your child's understanding or sympathy. If you are willing, however, to share your story because you want to care for and help your children, that is a great motivation and the conversation usually goes well.

Consider how Gary could have helped his son Scott by sharing his own childhood struggles. When Scott found the sexual videos at the video store, he was afraid of his own reaction. He was deeply troubled about all his sexual thoughts and feelings, yet he had to admit he was exhilarated by his fantasies. What would his dad have to say to him? How angry was he going to be? If Gary had been able to tell Scott about his own experiences as a preadolescent, Scott's confusion and loneliness probably would have been alleviated.

Maybe you're thinking that if your children know about your problems or struggles, it will give them permission to make their own mistakes. But every piece of research I have seen would indicate that when children have this kind of information, they are *less* likely to get in trouble with sexual sin. There is only one perfect parent, and that is God. Share you imperfections with your children. They will love you more for doing so.

Be Aware of How Your Own Story Affects You

Memories are powerful. Sometimes they are conscious; other times we are not aware of them and are very surprised when they surface. Watching your children go through the various stages of life can remind you of the struggles you faced at their age. Whatever feelings you experienced back then will surface and may catch you completely off guard. Many of our children's behaviors, words, or reactions have the ability to take us right back to our own childhood. This can be especially true with sexual behavior. Our children's sexual behaviors may remind us of times in our past that are painful.

When Gary heard that Scott had explored the sexually explicit video section, it took him right back to the time when his dad had punished him for the very same thing. The anger Gary felt had its roots in the past. Mostly, it wasn't about Scott or the fact that pornography was available at the video store. It was about how his father had handled a similar situation. As a young boy, Gary needed a loving father who could talk to him. That confrontation about pornography was probably not the only time that Gary's father punished him without talking to him, without helping him deal constructively with his feelings and behavior. When any of us are not given the emotional and spiritual nurturing we need, we are wounded

Gary has some grieving to do about what he didn't get from his father. He needs to express anger that his father's punishment was too harsh. Hundreds of men and women I have worked with have a "belt" story like Gary's. Spanking, when it does occur, needs to happen out of love and a desire to correct problem behavior. It should never be done in anger. Gary will need to experience healing for wounds created by his father's anger, forgive his dad for being human and making mistakes, and move on. Many incidents in his children's lives, like this one with Scott, will remind Gary of his need to do this healing work.

Gary is also afraid. He is legitimately afraid for his son because he knows the powerful effect pornography has had on his life. He doesn't want his son to fall victim to that power. The incident also reminds him of how much he was afraid of his own father. He needs to be able to talk to Kathy about these feelings and to other men who can support him.

Her children's experiences and behaviors also trigger memories for

Kathy. Her daughter's natural question left her speechless, not because she is incompetent as a mother, but because of her own sadness and the lack of modeling she received.

Kathy has another very real problem. Her sons' questions and behaviors are reminding her of the difficulty she and Gary are having sexually. Her distress comes not just from old memories but also from current painful realities. If she is not careful, she could take out her anger about Gary's behavior on her sons.

This story illustrates again why it is so important for you to talk to each other about sex in order to talk to your kids effectively. If Gary and Kathy can work on their own issues with their pasts and with each other, they will be a blessing to their children. Think of how much less afraid of their feelings children would be if they knew that their parents have experienced the same feelings and can model how to deal with them in a healthy way.

If you find yourself reacting strongly to your child's behavior, consider whether your own memories are surfacing. How old do you feel at that moment? Sometimes when we are trying to be a parent, our spirit is telling us that we are a child. Take care of that child. Get away from the situation for a few minutes. Talk to an adult who is able to be objective. Get advice and support. Allow the Holy Spirit to comfort you and help you discern what to say so that you can come back to being an adult with your child. Even if you have to miss the immediate opportunity to instruct your child, it is always better to talk after you have figured out where your feelings are coming from. It is never too late to have a conversation or to go back and redo or clean up a conversation that did (or didn't) happen earlier.

Use the Teachable Moment

When I was in high school, one of the girls in our church youth group got pregnant. In the sixties, of course, such situations were more unusual and definitely more shameful than they are today. My dad, her minister, found a place for her to go and have the baby. The child was then adopted. The girl eventually came back to school, but seemed distant, frightened, and depressed. I wanted to talk to her. I must confess, however, that alongside my genuine concern for her, I had sexual curiosity about how she had let this happen.

My dad talked to me about her situation. I don't remember all the things he said, but I do remember this: He said that she was no different from any of us who had ever had sexual temptations. He may have talked about the story of the woman caught in adultery, but I really don't remember. He simply said, "She needs a friend, one who will not judge her. Why don't you just treat her like you always have? Find a way to let her know that you are a safe friend." I still wasn't quite sure I knew how to do that, but I do remember making an effort to be a "safe" male for her. We remained friends until we graduated and went off to college.

My dad recognized a teachable moment when he saw one. By discussing a disconcerting situation with me at the right time, he gave me wise guidance and instilled values in me that directly influenced my behavior.

God presents parents with such opportunities all the time. During one brief afternoon at the mall, Gary and Kathy were presented with teachable moments about pregnancy, the use of sex appeal to sell products, sex appeal in general, and pornography. Quite a list. It's easy to feel overwhelmed as parents if we don't have much practice talking to our children about sex. If that is true in your family, you probably have a lot of corrective work to do. Relax. If you desire a lifetime of open conversations about sex, teachable moments will continue to come along, and you'll find it natural to keep the dialogue going.

Talk to Your Kids Together

As I have said, one of the best ways to model healthy sexuality is for parents to talk to their children as a team. The main dynamic we demonstrate by this is that a man and woman can talk *together* about this subject. We have often assumed that a father talks to a son and a mother talks to a daughter.

The potential problem with this logic is that women remain a mystery to boys and men remain a mystery to girls.

Earlier I described how Gary and Kathy might have talked to Molly about the subject of pregnancy. Again, this may seem like an overwhelming task if this is the first conversation they have had with her. Nevertheless, you see the principles at work: Gary and Kathy talk to each other first, coordinate their efforts, make Molly feel safe, and model to her that it is quite natural for a mom and dad together to talk about sex.

Admit Your Mistakes

All of these principles take practice. Be patient with yourself. Nobody is perfect. When you make a mistake, remember that you can teach your child a great principle of maturity by simply letting them know when you've been wrong. You are modeling taking responsibility for your own actions.

Let's imagine Gary and Kathy's scenario from a couple of different angles. First, let's assume that they didn't talk to any of their three kids about the experiences at the mall. It is five years later: Scott is sixteen, Matthew is eleven, and Molly is eight. Gary and Kathy realize they have made a mistake in not talking to them enough about sex (and maybe many other things). They could begin a conversation like this:

"We have asked to sit down and talk with you because we want to try to correct a situation in which we feel we've made a mistake. There are a number of things that we haven't talked to you about. One of those things is sex. We know that what we're about to talk about might be embarrassing. We won't talk long tonight. We won't put you on the spot. We may want to talk to each of you alone about some of these things. Hopefully, this is the beginning of many conversations. The main thing is that we want you to know we're fully aware that we're not perfect parents. There are reasons why it has been hard for us to talk to you about certain things, and we may explain some of those as we go along. For now, please accept our apology. We're going to try to do better."

The different ages of the children will dictate different parts of the conversation from this point, collectively and individually. My experience is that kids are resilient and forgiving. They will love you for your honesty.

Now let's consider a different scenario. Let's suppose that Gary has exploded at Scott out of his anger about the pornography. He has really shamed him and told him how perverted he is for looking at that "filth." Here's how he might start a conversation later:

"Son, I was really wrong to get angry with you. I'm sorry. I know I've hurt you, and I didn't mean to. I am asking for your forgiveness. I love you. You are a great and fine son. Looking at pornography is a very natural temptation for a boy your age. There is nothing wrong with you. There are several reasons why I got mad that have nothing to do with you. Those reasons are about me and the story of my life. If you're willing, I would like to tell you what those are. Most of all I want to help you avoid in your life some of the pain that I've experienced."

Gary is modeling several different things to his son. First, he is taking responsibility for his own actions. He is modeling confession and asking for forgiveness. He also is affirming his son. He is cleaning up old mistakes. Hopefully, he is also helping his son to feel less lonely and ashamed. On this foundation, Gary can start teaching Scott what he knows about controlling this kind of problem and begin sharing with Scott some of the lessons he's learned the hard way. Scott may have to learn some hard lessons too, but now his father will be an ally and not the enemy.

You may be wondering, "How can I admit my mistakes and still be the disciplinarian that I need to be? I won't have any credibility." Think about it this way: Who have you come to really respect in your life—those who always seem perfect and would never think of admitting to a mistake or those who do admit mistakes and have corrected or worked through them? I think most of us are more willing to submit to the authority of a humble person than to a self-righteous one.

You have seen how Gary and Kathy's children presented various questions and challenges according to their ages. The rest of this book examines five different age groups. As I've said, kids vary somewhat as to how they fit emotionally, physically, and spiritually into these divisions, so use them only as a general guide.

As you read, you may want to refer back to chapters 1–3 and review how to talk to each other, the model of healthy sexuality, and general principles for talking to your kids. This book is not meant to be read through just one time and then put on the shelf. In fact, I pray that you will meet with other parents, whose kids are roughly the same age as yours, and use this book as a discussion starter. Such a group could give you support and encouragement as you live through each stage of life with your kids.

CHAPTER FOUR

Infancy and Toddlerhood

(A G E   0 – 3)

At the age of three, Sarah was a typical walking, talking, increasingly independent little girl. She enjoyed putting long sentences together and was rather proud of herself. She had courageously confronted her fears of others and tolerated going to day care while her mom had a "morning out." Now it was time to finally master one of the great control issues of life: going to the bathroom on the toilet. Her parents had been very gentle, patient, and affirming as they reinforced the "big girl" behavior. Sarah was almost there. One day her older brother, John, forgot to close the bathroom door. As Sarah walked by and saw him, she was mystified. She ran to her mom and asked, "Why does John get to stand up when he goes to the bathroom?"

YOUR CHILD'S DEVELOPMENTAL TASKS

In order to develop normally, all children must master a number of developmental tasks. During the first three years of life, these tasks are very basic, but they begin to cement the foundation for healthy development throughout life. Hundreds of the people I counsel with who have sexual troubles later in life can trace some of their problems back to their earliest years. Therefore, healthy sexuality is built on the successful completion of the tasks in each stage of development.

Typically, healthy children will tackle the following tasks by age four:

- awareness of the body, its features and functions
- awareness that a person has a separate identity from others
- awareness of differences between male and female
- sense of being safe
- trusting self and trusting others
- courage to experiment on one's own
- eating
- talking
- walking
- control of bowels and bladder

Key words on this list include: *body, identity, control, safety,* and *trust.* The ability to know and like one's body, to be in control of its safety, to be comfortable with being male or female, and to be able to trust someone else are essential elements of healthy sexuality as we grow up and, ultimately, as we interact with a marriage partner.

YOUR PRIMARY PARENTING TASKS

In each of the five broad stages of your child's development, your tasks will be different in terms of helping your child develop healthy sexuality. In this early stage of your child's life, your tasks will involve meeting your child's basic needs and building his or her foundation for the future. You will see that the lessons and tasks of this stage are very simple and basic. They are, however, the foundation. Some psychologists say that 80 percent of what a person learns, he or she learns during this first phase of childhood.

Your tasks in this stage include:

- providing healthy touch
- responding consistently to your child's basic physical and emotional needs

- keeping your child safe while beginning to "let go"
- affirming your child's natural curiosity and sense of experimentation
- toilet training
- teaching basic skills
- providing information about differences of male and female. This may include information about where babies come from.

Think about the monumental importance of these tasks. Whenever possible, both parents should share the responsibility of carrying them out. It's important to stay calm and remember that God has built into most kids lots of resiliency when it comes to dealing with their parents' mistakes. Mistakes in this stage can be corrected by thoughtful and loving parents who seek and pray to do the right thing. As you go along, don't forget to talk to other parents who already have been through this stage. Always seek to be creative. Don't just rely on the parenting you received at various ages.

Now let's discuss these tasks in greater detail in light of the five dimensions of healthy sexuality.

HEALTHY SEXUALITY IN THE FIRST STAGE OF CHILDHOOD: PHYSICAL DIMENSION

Body Awareness

When babies are born, they are totally helpless. They must depend on their parents for everything. They don't have enough awareness even of themselves to know that they are separate human beings. In the first few months of life, they begin to become aware of their surroundings and of their own bodies. One of the main developmental tasks for a baby growing into a small child is to develop a sense of his or her own body and its abilities to interact safely with the environment. This means that babies will find out that they each have a body all to themselves, that it will be safely nurtured by others, and that there are certain things they can do on their own. They can control some of their bodily functions. They can learn to walk and to talk, rather monumental tasks when you stop to think about it.

As their eyes focus, babies recognize certain sights, most importantly the sight of their parents. As their ears develop, they will recognize the sound of their parents' voices. They experience that they don't like being cold or hot or wet. They certainly don't like to be hungry. The first way that they will learn how to get a response is to cry. Babies who don't experience consistent and loving responses to their crying in this stage may resort to crying throughout their childhood to get what they want. As their abilities to feel, hear, and see develop, they will get a sense that they are different and separate from the people who care for them.

Body Control

As children learn physical skills, they will begin to practice using them in a variety of ways. They will move their various body parts, discovering what each is capable of. They will start learning how to control their bladder and bowel functions. They will experiment with using their physical skills, especially as they become mobile, to find out how much power they have. They will try to understand what their ability to get around and be in rooms by themselves has to do with controlling their environment. Throughout all this experimentation, children learn powerful lessons about what they can and can't accomplish and get away with. These are experiments in limits, control, and self-will.

Jon was almost three years old. Toilet training was going well. He was really getting it. One day while on a picnic, Jon really had to go, but there were no toilets readily available. His dad took him off into the woods and showed him that it was possible to go close to the nearest tree.

Later that week, Jon and his mom were at the local mall. His mom was busy looking through some clothes on a rack, and Jon really had to go. He noticed a fountain with lots of small trees and shrubs around it and thought nothing of picking out one of those small trees to relieve himself on. He was really proud of himself. He had done what his dad showed him how to do.

Of course, Jon's mom was mortified. It is easy to imagine her anger and the possible results of it. She faced several unhealthy temptations. One was to simply take Jon and run. Another was to spank or somehow physically punish him with no explanation, telling him to never do that again. She could have simply shamed him by telling him in some fashion how stupid that was, again without explanation.

But as a healthy mom, she put Jon's action in perspective. She affirmed his sense of accomplishment. She did, however, begin instruction on healthy boundaries immediately, in this case by identifying the difference between public and private places.

"Jon, I'm proud of you for figuring out a place to go to the bathroom. You were doing what you and Dad did at the picnic the other day. I bet you thought you were being just like Dad, but we need to talk about the right places to do that and the wrong places."

The positive or negative nature of this kind of conversation will be primarily determined by the attitude of the parent. No matter what she says, if she is angry or embarrassed when she talks to her child, she will send the wrong message.

A child's basic early life experiences related to his bodily functions teach him about his body in ways that will be the foundation for later life experiences, including genital sexuality. If a child is affirmed about his body and how he controls it, then he will learn how to be independent and self-assured. If instead he is shamed, punished, or ignored as he experiments with using and controlling his body, then he may experience shame about himself and lack confidence in his ability to control how he interacts physically (including sexually) with the world around him.

Body Comfort

At twenty-seven, Michael was totally ashamed of himself. For years the only way he was able to go to sleep at night was to sexually fantasize and masturbate. He felt guilty about this but couldn't seem to stop. His wife was exasperated and blamed herself for not being sexually available enough.

Michael finally dragged himself to counseling. His Christian therapist helped him to trace this pattern back to his early years. He remembered the trouble he had sleeping when he was a little boy. Then it hit him. He remembered that when he was two and three years old, his mother would come into his room and massage his genitals. It felt nice and it relaxed him, and he went to sleep.

I don't think anyone would want to arrest Michael's mom for sexual abuse. She was doing what she thought necessary to get him to go to sleep. She may have been misinformed, naive, or maybe just repeating a pattern that had happened to her. The result, however, was an association between relaxing and genital touching that Michael learned to do for himself as he grew older. He will have to learn healthy forms of relaxation in order to break this pattern.

Can you see how important these early life experiences are? Part of the problem in Michael's case was that his mom was not touching him in other ways. She could have simply given him a backrub or held or rocked him. Today, even when Michael masturbates, what he really wants is loving touch.

It is common for babies to touch themselves in their genital areas. I have known parents who are horrified by this. They are embarrassed by it or think that it is somehow perverted. But at this stage a child's job is to explore himself and all of his bodily sensations. There is absolutely nothing wrong with this kind of touching. If, however, babies or small children are not getting healthy touch and nurture on other parts of their bodies from parents and other caregivers, they will begin to find substitutes. For some children, genital self-touching may be the only pleasurable touching they receive.

HEALTHY SEXUALITY IN THE FIRST STAGE
OF CHILDHOOD: EMOTIONAL DIMENSION

Trust

Babies and young children must have their needs met in consistent and dependable ways. This is not a matter of always giving them what they want; it is a matter of giving them what they need. Part of a child's task in this stage is to transition from crying about what he needs to being able to ask for it. A child doesn't know appropriate limits. It is up to parents to set consistent limits, not one thing one day and another the next. As parents provide consistent environments, bedtimes, meals, and clothing, a child learns to trust his parents.

How you handle your child's feelings during this stage is an important part of his learning to trust. In counseling, therapists often say to people, "Trust your feelings." It is okay to be sad, to cry, to be angry, to be frightened. Many people have been talked out of their feelings for years, however, with statements that often start in this stage of childhood. As a child, do you remember hearing your parents say things like "Big girls (or boys) don't cry"; "Don't make such a fuss"; "Now, now it doesn't really hurt"; "It's not okay for you to be angry like that (even though I'm being angry at you for being angry)"; or "God doesn't like it when you feel that way"?

It is normal for babies and young children to cry, have tantrums, and be frightened of the big world that they don't understand. It is crucial that parents reassure them, comfort them, and let them know that their feelings are normal.

Babies are also learning during this stage about who is "present" in their lives. They need to trust that both parents will be there for them. Perhaps one parent is working all the time or simply doesn't take time to be with, hold, or play with the child. The child will feel, even at this age, bereft of that parent's love and attention. This early sense of abandonment can present itself in a variety of ways later in life. What we will see in later chapters is that, given the presence of other influential factors, a child may learn to compensate for feeling abandoned and unloved. One way is to conclude that sexual activity is a way of getting attention and comfort.

Safety

As babies begin to learn motor skills, they will accomplish complicated gymnastics like rolling over, getting up on hands and knees, creeping along, and then crawling. There will come a dramatic day when a child first crawls into a room and realizes that he is alone. This can be extremely terrifying. Mom or Dad, of course, comes to rescue him. So he tries again and gets rescued again. Gradually, he learns to crawl away and then to crawl back to wherever Mom or Dad is. He crawls up and touches one of them on the leg, and then off he goes again. During this process, he is learning that it is okay to come and go and that someone will be there for him.

A parent's consistent and dependable presence is vitally important to a child's ability to trust and feel safe. What powerful creatures we parents are at this stage. How we handle that power, even during this early period, teaches our children about trusting our care, attention, and protection. Will we be there to meet their needs? Will we keep them safe? Children who do not get their basic needs met during this stage will have problems later with trusting and feeling safe in the world.

Recently I was talking to a woman who had major trouble trusting her husband when he was on business trips. She was convinced he was having an affair. The husband reassured me that he had never been unfaithful. As I questioned him about his behaviors, attitudes, and faith, it was obvious that he was telling the truth. Somewhere in his wife's past, her essential ability to trust and to feel safe with those who were supposed to love her had been damaged. You can see why the ability to trust and feel safe is so foundational to relationships and intimacy and, therefore, to sexuality.

HEALTHY SEXUALITY IN THE FIRST STAGE
OF CHILDHOOD: RELATIONAL DIMENSION

Individuation

When babies are first born, they don't have the ability to distinguish their identity from that of their parents'. They are enmeshed, particularly with the parent who holds, feeds, changes, and talks to them the most. Sometime during the first year of life, a baby begins to learn that he is separate from his mother and father. As he grows, this separation becomes more and more apparent. Much of the experimenting in a child's life is meant to accomplish this healthy separation.

Parents have their first experience with "letting go" when their child is about one year old. They must let go of their child's hands as he or she encounters the scary task of walking. Teaching your child how to walk is a paradigm for many physical and emotional skills to come. Parents must develop that sense of when to hang on and when to let go as their child goes through the many necessary phases of becoming a separate person.

Some parents are not good at encouraging their children to move beyond dependency. In many ways they like taking care of a baby, and so they continue to do things for a child long past the child's need to have them done. For some, parenting is a way to start over themselves. More than likely, the parent is lonely and finds comfort in the child's dependency. If the child tries to be independent, the parent will find a variety of ways to prevent the attempt.

One day your child will "walk" out the door on his or her first date or go to that first dance. How will you do then about letting them stumble and fall a few times? Trust is always a two-way process. You must do the work of helping your children to trust you. You also must teach them ways to be trustworthy. As they individuate from you and become more capable and responsible, you will need to let go at appropriate times. In this first stage of your child's life, you are practicing your skills as a parent just as much as your child is practicing his as a child.

Connecting

A child who has a hard time separating from a parent will have difficulty connecting to and giving himself to someone else. He might also have trouble being too dependent. A healthy marriage relationship is one in which both spouses have separate identities. Staying too enmeshed with each other is never healthy. All too often, one person who is dependent marries another who likes being depended on. You can imagine the variety of unhealthy dynamics that are possible in this scenario. How a parent relates to a child at ages one, two, and three will set the direction for how that child relates to others later, even well into adulthood.

Some parents are overly concerned about their child's safety. They worry incessantly and don't let their child experiment in the world for fear that he will somehow get hurt. Children who grow up in this kind of environment learn their parents' fears. Later, some will adopt a fearful stance themselves; others will throw caution to the wind and become rebellious. A rebellious child may have a hard time later submitting to the boundaries of an intimate relationship. A paranoid child will have difficulty taking the risks involved in living and loving fully.

The main point to remember about the relational dimension in this stage is that from their first relationship with their parents and other primary caregivers, children learn patterns of relating that will transfer to their later relationships, including marriage. Even though you will not be talking specifically with your children about the sexual relationship during this stage, you will be doing many things that will have a profound effect on their ability to have a healthy one later. Because having a healthy marriage depends on two spouses being whole individuals, being intimate friends, and having community outside of their relationship, you can see why proper development from birth to age three is so foundational. The ability to connect and trust and also to be separate and take risks is key to participating in healthy friendship and community.

HEALTHY SEXUALITY IN THE FIRST STAGE OF CHILDHOOD: PERSONAL DIMENSION

Gender Identity

One of the tasks of this stage of development is for a child to learn about gender difference. Boys are boys and girls are girls. Much of what we learn about the roles of boys and girls, men and women, are being formed even at this early age. Children see what mom and dad are doing, wearing, saying, and acting like. So, too, a child is observing all other boys and girls, men and women, in his or her environment.

Eli was three years old. He loved to play with Jessica, also three, who lived across the street. Jessica had three older sisters, and her dad wasn't home very much. The main people she knew were girls. In that certain knowledge, she did her best day by day to convince Eli that he, too, was a girl. She would insist that Eli play with dolls. No matter what Eli was wearing, she would want him to dress up in some of her clothes. Eli came home one day really confused and said to his mom, "Why am I a boy? Jessica says that I'm really a girl."

This situation needs special attention. Eli's world must be kept safe. His parents will need to talk to Jessica's parents so they can address this issue with her. If she does not change, play with her should be stopped, as hard as this might be. The main priority is to maintain safety for Eli.

It is critical to help a child establish a correct sense of gender identity. Eli's parents will need to talk to him about the difference between boys and girls. Age-appropriate picture books, even for two- and three-year-olds, will show him the anatomical differences between boys and girls. Some of these books are listed in the resource section.

The following conversation is an example of the simple nature of the message that needs to be reaffirmed over and over to children. Notice that there is a biblical message (Psalm 139) paraphrased in it.

"Eli, you are such a big boy now. You know that God made you and that you are very special. He made you to be a boy. Let me show you a book that has some pictures that will help you understand. You see, boys have a penis. Girls have a vagina. Your dad has a penis just like you. Your mom has a vagina. Jessica was wrong in what she told you. I don't know why she said what she did. Maybe she was confused or just wanted you to be a girl like her sisters. But you are a boy. From the very first day that God made you, he made you in a wonderful way to be a boy. He has very special plans for you, and as you grow up, he will help you to know what those are. Being a boy is very special. God has made all of us different in many ways. I'm really glad that you were able to come to me and tell me about this situation. This must have been really scary and confusing for you."

In later chapters I will discuss sexuality problems that can develop later in life, such as homosexuality, gender confusion (being born female and thinking that you're really male or vice versa), cross-dressing, and others. All have their roots in wounds experienced during this early stage. If these kinds of problems do in fact begin this early, that could be one reason why most people who have them don't remember making a choice about how they feel and behave. If Eli didn't get the proper affirmation and correction from his parents in this situation, he might internalize his confusion and be vulnerable to problems later.

HEALTHY SEXUALITY IN THE FIRST STAGE OF CHILDHOOD: SPIRITUAL DIMENSION

Being a parent is an awesome responsibility. One of the reasons it is so hard for me is because I recognize that my role as father will influence my children as they try to understand God as Father and Jesus as Lord.

Sarah, the little girl in our opening story, seemed to be developing normally in every way. One night her mother sat down by her bed and said to her, "Let's say our prayers and talk to Jesus." Sarah replied, "I don't want to talk to Jesus." Her mother was horrified and didn't know what to say. Very matter-of-factly Sarah continued, "I don't think that Jesus likes me. He's not my friend. He never comes over to our house. I've never seen him. When I talk to him he doesn't answer me. Grandma and Grandpa come over. My friends come over. You and Daddy talk to me. Why doesn't Jesus come over to my house and talk to me?"

Although psychologists might tell us otherwise, even small children can be logical thinkers. This little girl thought in rather black-and-white terms. How her parents begin to explain to her the existence and the mystery of the living Christ is important, but not easy. In Luke 18:17 Jesus said, "I tell you the truth, anyone who will not receive the kingdom of God like a little child will never enter it." I think Jesus knew that young children are naturally very trusting. He was instructing us that we must come to God with childlike trust. Helping your children develop the ability to trust in you as earthly parents is the first crucial step in teaching them to trust in the spiritual dimension.

Little Sarah did trust the key people in her life. So over the years she will come to understand that Jesus is with her in many ways that she can't see. If her parents are wise, they won't try to talk her out of her feelings and black-and-white thinking; instead, they will try to reframe things for her. They will try to teach her that her mom and dad, grandma and grandpa, and friends are part of a larger family that is God's family. Maybe a conversation with Sarah will go like this.

"You know that we often talk to you about God, his Son Jesus, and the Holy Spirit. It is always hard to understand something that you can't see. It is hard to know about someone if you haven't seen them. It is really hard to understand that God made you, every inch, and that you are precious to him.

"Think about your friend Jane: She is not here now, is she? You saw her yesterday. If there were someone here now who had never seen Jane, how would you tell him that Jane is alive? You have a picture of her in your mind. You know what she is like. You would explain that Jane is your friend. You like her. She likes you. Those feelings are in your heart. It's the same way with God and Jesus. Some people who were alive long ago actually saw him. They wrote about him in the Bible, and the Bible tells us that he still lives today. There are many thousands and millions of other people who know that Jesus is alive today because they know about him in their hearts.

"Dad and I love each other even at times when we are not together and can't see each other. We love Jesus even though we have never seen him either. We know in our hearts that he is with us. We are trying to tell you about him even now. And our love for you is a part of God and Jesus loving you. And they love you in such better ways than even we can. As you grow older, we hope and pray that you will come to know God and Jesus as we do."

Sarah will have lots of other questions and misgivings as she grows, just as we all do. That is a natural part of growing in faith. But a child's ability to trust is often so pure that she will believe something if we tell her it is true.

As Sarah grows, she will recall many of the messages that she accepted as a little girl. As her body changes, she will need to know that this is part of God's design for her. As she questions her appearance, she will need to remember that God made her—fearfully and wonderfully. As she wonders about relationships, she will need to remember that Jesus is her friend and that there are many others in her family and circle of friends who love her too. As she meets boys and finds one that she wants to marry and be sexual with, she will need to remember how her mom and dad modeled the importance of committing that marital relationship to Christ.

See how important your job is as a model and teacher of spiritual truth? It is indeed an awesome task, but it is one of the great privileges and joys of parenting.

HEALTHY SEXUALITY CHECKLIST

By age four, a child will have put in place some foundational building blocks. While we can't expect small children to fully understand something like genital sexuality, we can help them from birth onward to understand themselves and their bodies in a way that will be a solid foundation for developing healthy sexuality as they grow older.

Here's a brief summary of the points we've covered in this chapter as they relate to the model of healthy sexuality.

Physical. Children will learn that they have separate bodies that can feel and move. They will learn how to walk and talk and be toilet trained. They will experience getting their physical needs met, not just because they cry, need to be fed, or need to be protected, but because they are loved. Most of all they will be held, rocked, soothed, and nurtured in safe ways. Children will also learn about safety, healthy control, power, and proper boundaries in all of their physical activities.

Emotional. At this time children are too young to understand complex emotions, but their parents can establish a foundation by teaching that it is safe to be sad, angry, frightened, or lonely and that their parents or caregivers will deal with these emotions in responsible, consistent, and dependable ways. The primary task of this stage is to help children know how to trust themselves, their bodies, and their emotions, as well as how to trust others. Trust is the foundation of relationship and intimacy and is, therefore, the foundation of healthy sexuality.

Relational. Children will discover that they are part of a larger family. They will learn that they can be independent and have control over certain aspects of themselves but that certain limits and boundaries must be respected. In addition to learning to trust the people around them, they will practice acting independently and connecting to others besides their parents.

Personal. Children will know the difference between boys and girls and have a clear identity as male or female. Healthy male and female characteristics and roles will be modeled for them.

Spiritual. Children should be taught that they have a heavenly Father and that God made them and loves them in very special ways. They will begin to understand that when the people who love them, including God, are not with them physically, those people can still be counted on for love and support. In this way, they begin to develop the building blocks of faith.

CHAPTER FIVE

Childhood

(A G E   4 – 9)

Elizabeth, age seven, recently asked her mother if she could wear a "grown-up" night-gown to bed instead of the pajamas that she had always worn as a "little girl." After several nights of doing this and feeling so proud of herself, she decided that she didn't need to wear underwear either. Feeling very grown up, she came downstairs to tell her dad goodnight. Enthusiastically she announced to her dad and her five-year-old brother, Andrew, that she had something to show them. With that she pulled up her nightgown to show them both that she wasn't wearing anything underneath.

Elizabeth's dad was both shocked and amused. Andrew was curious and started to reach over to touch the private parts of his sister that she'd proudly put on display.

This brief story illustrates this stage of life for children. They naturally are proud of accomplishments, just as Elizabeth was. They also are naturally curious and will explore their world, just as Andrew did.

YOUR CHILD'S DEVELOPMENTAL TASKS

In early childhood, kids change very rapidly in terms of their physical appearance and proficiencies. There will be a wide variation in physical development, particularly in the seventh through ninth year. During that time, it is even possible for girls to enter puberty and begin menstruating and manifest other forms of physical sexual development. (If your daughter experiences early onset of puberty, you'll find material pertinent to this in the next chapter.)

Parents need to understand that even children as young as four to six can have a wide range of sexual feelings, from pleasurable feelings in the genital area to a preoccupation with various parts of the body or bodily function. It is known that even male babies have erections; this is a normal part of their physical chemistry.

Sexual curiosity and experimentation are normal during this stage. The foundation for healthy sexuality continues to be built as parents help guide their children through the key developmental tasks they face between the ages of four and nine. The key word is *foundation*. Many of the things I will talk about in this chapter may not always seem to pertain directly to sexuality. Remember the broad nature of our sexuality model. All of the dynamics discussed either directly relate to sexuality or they are building the foundation for later years. Here is a brief list of your child's developmental tasks between the ages of four and nine:

- understand his or her body, how it functions, and the early essentials of self-care
- understand the basic biology of sex and reproduction
- begin to learn how to honestly express emotions
- become aware of unhealthy ways to use behaviors or substances as emotional coping strategies
- explore male and female social relationships and friendship
- understand appropriate social boundaries
- experience the home as a safe place
- understand how to maintain the safety of his or her own body
- develop a personal conscience and a sense of what is morally right and wrong

YOUR PRIMARY PARENTING TASKS

Children today are being exposed more and more to sexually explicit material at young ages, and they will be naturally curious about it. Sadly, my experience would even suggest that the number-one place kids discover pornography for the first time is through their parents' collection. Even if that is not the case, the covers of our most popular magazines are getting more and more pornographic. Many public places, like supermarkets, have these available at the eye level of our children. Also, schools are doing a wonderful job of educating kids about using computers. Most of them are more computer literate than we are. If we have access to the Internet on our home computers, it will be another potential source of extreme danger to kids in this age group.

As a parent you are going to have to deal with complex sexual issues much earlier today than may have been the case a number of years ago. A part of your spirit may rebel against having to talk to your kids about specific sexual practices, but if you don't, you will have to keep them away from TV, radio, movies, magazines, and newspapers. Such restrictions will make them feel totally isolated, and the harm of that at this age is devastating.

Talking to your children about sex early does not mean you're conforming to the pattern of the world; it means you are preparing your children for the inevitable battles they ultimately will have to wage in their own lives. You are giving them the ammunition for renewing their minds.

In this second stage of your child's life, your tasks will include:
- monitoring and supervising all of your child's activities
- instructing him or her in basic biology
- providing opportunities to interact socially
- providing safety in your home
- recognizing the emotional roots of certain behavioral problems
- helping your child process feelings

• instructing him or her in God's moral design

• affirming him or her emotionally, physically, and spiritually

I'm aware that lists like these can feel overwhelming. Remember to take a break and be gentle with yourself, to provide yourself with good self-care, to talk to each other, and to find support as parents.

HEALTHY SEXUALITY DURING EARLY CHILDHOOD: PHYSICAL DIMENSION

Curiosity

Luke was a naturally inquisitive six-year-old. One day when his older sister walked by, he lifted up her dress to see what was underneath. Luke's mom was horrified and slapped Luke's hand with the wooden spoon she was cooking with. When Luke cried from the pain, she said simply, "Don't ever do that again!" End of discussion.

Luke's mother was continually afraid that one of her children would do something wrong, and she believed it was her job to punish them severely. She was especially vigilant in the area of sexuality. We can only imagine what the negative environment of that home was like. Such an atmosphere will not only kill a child's natural sense of curiosity and wonder, but also will infuse his early ideas about sexuality with shame and fear.

One of the keys to all of our conversations with our kids during this stage will be to affirm our child's natural investigative activities and his or her sense of curiosity. We will never want to discourage that. A child will need that sense of discovery and enthusiasm in so many other of life's activities.

From three years old and on, walking is very natural for children. They will run all over with great grace and ease. They have also mastered talking in complete sentences and will exercise that skill regularly. The ability to be verbal also signals that a child is being verbal with himself. At this age, children begin the "internal dialogue" that will be a running conversation for the rest of their lives. The ability to get around and to talk to others and to oneself combine to give a child the ability to explore his or her world and to begin to imagine all the possibilities of what it could be like. It is a stage of adventure, role-playing, excitement, and tremendous energy.

The energy of this stage will lead children to be naturally aggressive and to continue to explore the nature of their physical powers and sensations. How we encourage or discourage this will be vital during this stage.

Pat, age six, was playing with her cousin Beth, age seven, who was visiting for the summer. Since they were so young, they often slept in the same bed. They had discovered that it felt good to touch each other's vagina. One night when they were in bed, Beth said, "Do you want to do something that I saw my older sister doing?" Pat said, "Sure," and Beth proceeded to climb on top of her and bounce up and down. When Pat's parents discovered this, they didn't know what to think.

This story is not about two little girls who will become lesbians. It is first and foremost about curiosity and play. It is also about sex. It needs to be treated for what it is and to be handled with respect.

Pat's mom asked her niece, "Beth, where did you learn to do that?" Beth said she had seen her sister and her boyfriend doing that and it seemed like fun. For the time being, the mom talked to the girls about private parts of their body and said that they would need to talk more tomorrow. She said, "Is it all right if we talk about this later? I promise I will talk to you more about what you saw, Beth." The girls were fine with this.

The next day she called her sister, Beth's mom, and asked her what information she had shared with Beth about sex. "Nothing," her sister responded. "Beth is too young for that."

Boys and girls in this age group are very curious about the differences between male and female. It is common to find them asking each other, "Show me yours and I will show you mine." Sex play as children, the proverbial "playing doctor," is a common fact of life. Remember that kids in this stage are naturally curious and they will experiment. They want to find out how they are alike and different from each other. Parents need to know that this is experimentation with anatomy and not necessarily with genital sex. Avoid overreacting. Don't assume that this is a dangerous situation. Such an occasion provides the opportunity to review safe boundaries and private areas of the body, but it is also a time to affirm their curiosity. Addressing specific anatomical questions will also be necessary. Children will need to know about the vagina, vulva, penis, testicles, and erections. Intercourse can ultimately be explained as a wonderful picture of how God created us to become "one flesh." There is always a lesson about God's design that can be included in these conversations.

When we parents encounter sex play, we must be careful to send the right messages to our curious children. Pat's mom will need to talk to her sister about what happened and how she would like to handle it. In this situation an aunt will become the designated giver of appropriate information. Beth's mom has a lot of soul-searching to do and will need to continue this conversation when Beth gets home. She also will have a lot of talking to do with her older daughter about the sexual nature of her relationship with her boyfriend.

The next day, Pat's mom sat down with both Pat and Beth. She showed them a cartoon book that described sex and gently explained to the girls what this was about. She also told them that sex is something that happens between a husband and wife.

"Beth, your sister is wrong to be having sex with her boyfriend. That is something that God wants us to wait for marriage to do. Your mom will have to talk to her about that. It is a mistake that many of us make. Your sister is not a bad person for doing this, but she will need to think about not having sex until she gets married. As for you two, it is natural to experiment with things like this. I completely understand why you are curious about it. Parts of our bodies, like our vaginas, feel good when they are touched. That is not a bad thing. But again, that is something reserved for the love that exists between a husband and wife. You two should not be touching each other there. Your vaginas are private parts and should not be shared with anyone else until you get married."

Pat's mom is taking the healthy approach. These two girls are getting love, attention, affirmation, and appropriate information. Luke, in the other story, got the opposite. With experiences like this, Pat and Beth are likely to have normal sex lives when they grow up. Luke, on the other hand, may have some sexual dysfunctions, particularly if that experience with his mother is indicative of many others in his growing-up years.

Imagine, for example, what his mom's reaction communicates to Luke about his general sense of awe and wonder about sex. In his marriage, if his wife were ever to say no to sex, for whatever reason, her response might take him right back to situations like this one. Also, Luke may develop deep anger with his mom if this is the way she normally handles his sexual curiosity. If he is not careful, he could take out that anger on his wife. I talk to many wives who can't understand why their husbands get so angry about sexual things in general. Chances are, their reactions go back to childhood experiences like Luke's.

If Luke's mom, on the other hand, had affirmed him for being curious and *then* (timing is everything) taught him about appropriate boundaries with his sister, the whole situation would have been different. Calm and loving tones are also much more helpful than shouts and shaming. Luke's mom could go back and correct this situation by first admitting her mistake, as we talked about in chapter 3, and then continuing with affirmation and loving correction.

Masturbation

Marcia, age eight, loved the feeling of the rushing water in the bathtub and came to discover that it was especially pleasurable when it touched her genital area. She had learned to position herself in such a way that it would increase this sensation. The more she experimented with this, the better at it she got. She also discovered that she could achieve the same sensation when she touched herself there. One day, her mom came into her bedroom to help her get ready and discovered Marcia doing this.

A child who is naturally inquisitive will explore his or her own body and be aware of those feelings that are pleasurable. Marcia is normal. Self-touching at these early ages is not about genital sexuality, at least in terms of its sexual content. Like so many of the situations we have dealt with, one of the dangers is that we might overreact. When that happens, the sense of shame a child will feel can be profound. This shame about their bodies can have a negative effect later in life. Fortunately, Marcia's mother was wise in her response.

"It feels good to touch yourself there, doesn't it?" Marcia's parents had already talked with her a number of times about sex, so it was natural for her mom to continue this conversation now. "I don't want to embarrass you by talking about this at length, so let me just say that the main reason it feels good to touch yourself like you were doing is because that area of your body will feel very good when you have sex with your husband. That is the way God designed a woman's body. There are just two things I want to say to you now about it, and we can talk more if you want to, now or later. First, just like sex, something like this is very private and should never be done with anyone else until you are married. Second, sometimes a person can get so used to doing this that it can get out of control."

This is not the end of their conversation. Many things about masturbation have been left unsaid. But these comments are enough for now. Too much information can overwhelm a child this age. Marcia's mother has done some important work, however. She has dealt with a potentially embarrassing situation for her daughter in a very nonshaming way. She has helped her daughter know that she is normal. Finally, she has left the door open and laid a foundation for future discussion about this issue and others.

The Biology of Sex and Reproduction

One night Patsy, age five, went into her brother Adam's room and climbed up on his bed. When her mom discovered her, she asked Patsy what she was doing. The little girl very seriously replied, "I'm counting his ribs. I need an extra one to make myself a sister."

This is one of those teachable moments. It is not just the message that only God can do this kind of orthopedic surgery. It is a time to talk about the fact that God made male and female as an integral part of his creation. It is also a time to talk about where babies, like sisters, really come from.

Patsy's mom and dad discussed how to approach their first conversation with their daughter about intercourse, pregnancy, and childbirth. They knew that they couldn't be too technical at this age, but that they needed to cover the basics. They also knew that Patsy, at her age, would need to see some pictures in order to understand what her parents were talking about. They bought a book (listed in the resource section) titled Where Did I Come From? *They liked the book because it used cartoon characters to give the general idea without being graphically specific.*

Together all three of them sat on the couch and read through the book. Patsy's parents started the conversation by saying, "We're going to talk to you about some things we've never talked about before. The other day you were thinking about making a baby. We'd like to explain how babies are really made." Patsy's parents treated this very naturally, and Patsy didn't seem to be embarrassed. They went through all of the pictures, and Patsy was very interested.

Patsy had some basic questions. "Does it hurt to have sex?" she asked. The book had already talked about the fact that it didn't, but she needed to hear it from her parents. They both reassured her. Patsy was also curious about how often it happened. Her mom and dad told her that it happens differently for different couples. How often husbands and wives have sex is something that they like to talk about by themselves. Patsy's dad said, "You know when you have your friend Jessica over to play, you sometimes whisper things to each other. You have secrets that are a part of your very special friendship. That doesn't mean that you don't love us or others. Well, Mom and I are like that, too. We have our very special secrets that are just between us. That has nothing to do with how much we love you."

Patsy's bottom-line question was, "Well, will you make me a baby sister?" Her par-

ents chuckled and told her that they were praying about whether to have another child. They said that if it was in God's plan for their family, they would. Then Patsy's mom said to her, "You really want a sister, don't you? Tell us why." Patsy said she just thought it would be fun to have a playmate.

The goal of conversation during this stage is to present basic facts, illustrate them in ways kids can comprehend, and then let the conversation proceed into related areas. Patsy's mom and dad let her dictate the direction in which the conversation went, and they calmly and naturally responded to her specific questions. Now, in later conversations, even if Patsy talks to just one of her parents about specific sexual issues, she knows that both of her parents are able to talk to her and that they talk to each other. This is vital modeling.

The question of how old is old enough to hear about the biology of genital sexuality is a highly controversial subject, particularly in the Christian community. Many parents are afraid that if they tell their kids about sex, they will be sexual. On the contrary, every piece of research I have seen suggests that the less kids know about sex, the more likely they are to experiment with it. Not knowing about sex increases the mystery.

Seven-year-old Amy is inquisitive. Her natural sense of wonder has always been a joy to all and helps her do well in school. When Amy's mom and dad explained the fundamentals of sex to her and where babies come from, they showed her a picture book that used cartoon characters to portray the basics of sex in nongraphic form. The book also explained pregnancy and where babies come from.

Amy took it all in with wide eyes but was not satisfied. She said, "Mom, do you and Dad have sex like that?" When her mom said yes, Amy's next question was, "Well, then, I would really like to see that. Can I watch? I won't say anything. I'll just sit in the corner."

Amy's mom and dad will have to refrain from being horrified and from laughing. Mature parents will recognize that this is a perfectly natural request from an inquisitive child and that it should be handled respectfully. Here's what Amy's parents said.

"Amy, you really like to see things for yourself, don't you? God has given you a wonderfully inquisitive mind. You need to understand that having sex is something that a husband and wife do and that it is a very special activity between them. It is about the love they feel for each other, and it is so special that it is meant to be enjoyed by them in private. It is only for them and is a part of the beauty, just between them, of their marriage. So no, you can't watch. Someday when you're married, you and your husband will have this special relationship, and you won't want anyone else to enjoy it but you."

These are wise parents. They responded calmly and as a couple. They affirmed Amy and didn't overreact to her question. They relied on an appropriate picture book to illustrate the basics. They taught her the correct moral message. Amy is a fortunate girl. If this experience is typical of those that take place in her house, she is much more likely to wait for sex until God shows her the right man to marry.

My belief is that kids in this age group need to know the basic biology of sex in terms that they can understand. They don't need the discussion to be graphically specific or extensive, but they do need to have the information. The challenge is to find a balance between no information and too much information. As a parent, it is your job to provide this information, rather than leaving the task to the school, the church, or your child's peer group. Don't wait for your child to verbalize what may be going through his or her mind, but don't try to mind read either. This stage may be one of those times to tell your own story.

Amy's mom decided to continue the conversation with her about sex. She began, "You know, I remember when I first heard what sex was all about. One of the girls at school told me about it and acted like I was dumb because I didn't already know.

I thought it sounded pretty horrible. I didn't like boys much at all. All the ones that I knew at school were pretty awful. I didn't like the idea of anything being inside me. I worried that it would hurt. I sometimes wished that I were a boy. They seemed to get to do more things.

"When I got older, I started liking boys. At first that surprised me. It will probably happen to you in a few years too. Then I met your dad and fell in love with him and wanted to get married and have kids. Even then God knew about you and that you would be a special gift to us. I still worried about sex. But it wasn't at all like what I worried about. It really feels nice, just like the picture book said. I know it's hard to wonder about all of these things until you get married, but I can only tell you it's really worth the wait."

What a wonderful gift this mom gave her daughter—the honesty of herself. I imagine that this kind of conversation is only one of many. When Amy's mom talks like this, she gives Amy the freedom, when she does have specific concerns and feelings, to share them with her mom or her dad. These parents are creating safety for the process of their daughter's sexual development.

Ben was four and the only one in the family who had red hair. His parents and his older brother and sister were all blonds. People loved his hair. Many times in an effort to be cute, some people teased him by asking how he got that hair when both his parents are blonds. Then they would tell him a joke that he was much too young to understand, "Maybe the mailman brought it." The next time Ben was asked the question, "Where did you get that hair?" he responded, "In the mailbox."

Ben is wondering why he is different from the rest of his family. Even though everyone around him seems to love his red hair, he may come to hate it because it sets him apart. Ben is too young to understand complicated genetics and the fact that red hair is a recessive genetic trait, but he is not too young to have the basic biology of sex and pregnancy explained to him.

Ben's parents bought a book about sex and pregnancy, illustrated with cartoon characters. They planned a very special outing for him and took him to the park. They all had a fun time playing, swinging on the swings, throwing a ball, running, and laughing. Along the way they pointed out every bird, every insect, every flower, every plant, every tree.

At one point Ben's dad said, "Ben, do you see how many different kinds of bugs, birds, plants, and trees God has created for us? God does that in a very special way. All of this comes from seeds that are planted in various ways. Do you remember when we planted the flower seeds in the pot and you watered it and a flower grew? There are lots of ways that seeds can be planted. Babies grow from seeds that come from a father and grow inside of a mother. I have a book here that shows how that happens. If you'd like to read it together, we can. But first I want to remind you how special you are to God and to your mom and me.

"You know, your red hair is like all of the colors out here in the park. It is part of God's rainbow. It is special just like you are. Even I can't really understand why some people have blond or black or brown or red hair. God meant for you to be a redhead. Everyone loves your hair. I hope that you will too."

Ben will now read through the book with his mom and dad. This will take time, and it may be something they look at often. Initially, a child can be frightened by this information. A boy may wonder about his penis being big enough for something like this to happen. Girls, like Patsy in our earlier story, may have a hard time with the idea of something being inside of them. A girl may wonder why she doesn't have a penis, and somewhere in her mind the idea of genital sexuality might seem like an invasion.

Do you see why it is crucial for mom and dad to talk together with their children about these things? Remember that your attitude often is more important in the conversation than specific information. If you are negative about sexuality, or if you are afraid of it, or if you have unresolved issues with sex, having a conversation about the biology of sex will be hard. Remember, attitude, attitude, attitude.

HEALTHY SEXUALITY DURING EARLY CHILDHOOD:
EMOTIONAL DIMENSION

At age seven, Mike discovered that at times his penis got bigger and harder, and this frightened him. He didn't know what it meant. Strangely, to him, it also felt rather good, so he would touch himself to increase his sense of pleasure. This felt somehow "bad" to him, but he wondered how something that was bad could also feel so good. It brought him comfort and calmed him down whenever he was feeling anxious or lonely.

As we discussed in the physical dimension, self-touching at this age is a normal part of a child's exploration of his body. It can become a problem, however, if it becomes repetitive in an obsessive way, a substitute for healthy nurture, or a coping mechanism for a child who does not know how to deal with his emotions.

Mike started touching his penis often and sometimes wasn't even aware that he was doing it. It was not uncommon for one of his parents to walk into the TV room and find him rather expressionless and "zoned out," watching TV with his hand down the front of his pants.

If a child is using self-touching as a form of comfort, it becomes necessary to try to understand what the child needs comforting about. A child who is obsessively masturbating may simply need to learn other solutions to dealing with his feelings about normal life problems.

Mike's dad talked to him one day when he discovered Mike masturbating in front of the TV. "You know most boys your age begin to discover how good it feels to touch themselves like you were doing just now. If you're like me when I was your age, you may not always know that you're doing this. At other times, though, I bet that you do know and that you enjoy the sensations it brings. I don't want to embarrass you, but if it's okay, I'd like to talk about a couple of things.

"First, you need to be careful about doing that in public. Other people can get embarrassed or offended when they see that. It's just not commonly accepted social

behavior. Second, have you heard the word masturbation?*" Mike had heard some of his friends tease about it but wasn't going to admit it. "Well,* masturbation *is a word used to describe rubbing your penis in such a way that you experience that pleasurable feeling. As you get older and your body changes, when you do that you can actually cause yourself to ejaculate, like you would if you were having sexual intercourse.*

"Many people, both boys and girls, experiment with masturbation, and we'll talk more about it as you grow older. For now, one thing concerns me. I don't know if you can answer this question now, but I wonder if you ever notice that you do this when you are worried about something, when you're angry, sad, or maybe bored. Think about that, and let's talk some more about this later."

Mike's dad is not pushing the issue, and I'm sure that Mike will be glad when his dad is done talking about this subject. The door to conversation, however, has been opened. If nothing else, a seed has been planted in Mike's mind that may help him become more self-aware and conscious of the feelings that might underlie his behavior. Mike's dad also has modeled to him that he is willing to talk about such things and that there is no shame in doing so.

Remember that the emotional dimension of healthy sexuality hinges on the ability to honestly express feelings. Self-touching is only one of the many behaviors or substances that kids this age may use to mask, avoid, or deal with feelings that are too confusing or frightening. Following is a partial list of some other behaviors to watch for that might indicate your child needs help developing emotionally:

- too much TV
- playing electronic games
- being overly absorbed with the computer
- overeating
- not eating
- being overly involved in any game or activity
- isolating
- obsession with one friend
- violent or disruptive behavior

Using sex, food, and other things to cope with emotions begins even at this age and can continue throughout life unless help is sought. If you suspect that your child is using a particular behavior to cope with his feelings, reread the section on the emotional dimension of sexuality in chapter 2 and consider some of the things you can do to help your child process feelings. Remember, the best thing you can do is to model emotional health by talking to your child about your own feelings and showing him or her that it is safe to do so.

Mike's dad added a couple of other things before he wrapped up the conversation. "Before I finish, let me just tell you that when I was your age I used to do this too. One day, my mom—your grandma—found me doing it. Was she ever angry! She told me that all kinds of bad things were going to happen to me if I kept doing it. She told Grandpa later, and he spanked me. I felt terrible. Well, I kept doing it for a while and none of those bad things happened, and I did it more and more often.

"I was really lonely and frightened and didn't think I had anyone to talk to. When I brought myself pleasure by touching my penis, it made me feel better. But what I really wanted and needed was someone to understand me and assure me that all of the different things I was feeling were okay to talk about.

"I just hope that if you ever feel like that, you'll be able to talk to me. I love you, Son, and I'm always here for you."

In the months and years ahead, as Mike's dad follows through in his commitment to being available and compassionate with his son, Mike will discover that his internal emotional terrain is not something to be frightened about or to avoid. Rather than using masturbation or any other activity to escape his feelings, he will be more likely to talk about them and develop emotionally. Hopefully he will also learn to identify what he really wants and needs.

HEALTHY SEXUALITY DURING EARLY CHILDHOOD: RELATIONAL DIMENSION

Friendship

Socially, boys and girls interact very comfortably at these ages, although cultural influences may teach them that they're not supposed to like each other. Much of the energy and curiosity of this stage can be used to explore play and friendship. Although we traditionally think that adolescence is the first time that boys and girls discover real friendship with each other, it's more true that they have been friends all along. Playing, cooperating, and learning together are parts of this stage. When adolescence begins, other powerful sexual urges and emotional feelings enter the mix and begin to make friendship more challenging.

During this stage one of our parental tasks is to provide opportunities for boys and girls to interact socially. Children should not be isolated, and boys and girls should have many opportunities to interact. This helps dispel the idea that the opposite sex is a great mystery. School, church, and sports are some of the main places that social interaction can take place at this stage. These activities should be supervised by those who can help kids talk to each other in productive ways.

I once worked as a volunteer in a fourth-grade class to help the kids understand the dangers of drugs. They participated in a variety of exercises that helped them talk to one another. I distinctly remember how, during one of these exercises, a group of boys was compelled to talk with a group of girls about some of their feelings about sports and competition. The girls created a skit, which included a dance that humorously portrayed the boys in a competitive situation on the basketball court. It was wonderfully funny and very healing for all of them. Experiences like this will help boys and girls be less competitive and less frightened of each other. This is a great lesson for later dating, romance, friendship, and marriage.

In addition to creating opportunities for opposite-sex interaction, adults need to model for kids how to appreciate the differences between males and females. God made the sexes different, and all of what God makes is good. If we understand and affirm each other, we can complement each other.

Social Boundaries

During this stage, children continue to learn that they are part of a larger community—first their family, then their church or school and peer group. Whether the setting is day care, preschool, or kindergarten, children will be learning the rules of acceptable behavior outside the home. Many of these may be the same as in the home, but now other adults will enter a child's world to model and teach them about the rules.

Many teachable moments present themselves during this stage. Remember the story about Elizabeth and her brother that opened this chapter? How would you handle this situation? Andrew and Elizabeth's dad sat them both down and had this chat.

"Elizabeth, we're very proud of you for being such a big girl that you are wearing nightgowns now. Andrew is very curious to see anyone who is different than he is. You are both different and very special to God. You two are different from each other because you're a girl, Elizabeth, and you, Andrew, are a boy. Mom and I are so happy that God gave us each of you.

"Both of you need to learn that certain parts of our bodies are private, and at certain times and places people can be embarrassed if we were to show them what the private parts of our bodies look like. A girl's vagina and a boy's penis are private parts of your body. Elizabeth, later when you get bigger and have breasts like Mom does, those are private parts also. Can either of you think of being any place in public when you've

seen people show these private parts? We also need to respect others and not ask to see them or ask to touch them. Do you both understand?"

This brief conversation may suffice for the moment. Notice the balance between affirming the children and stating boundaries in simple terms. Elizabeth or Andrew might ask why people are so embarrassed. It is a good question, especially when neither one of them felt particularly embarrassed by the situation. This fact underscores that one of a child's tasks during this stage is to learn what his or her environment and culture is comfortable with and not comfortable with. This is the beginning of social awareness and appropriateness that will be extremely important later.

HEALTHY SEXUALITY DURING EARLY CHILDHOOD: PERSONAL DIMENSION

The homes in which we live must be sanctuaries for our children as they grow. I love the word *sanctuary*, not just because I have been in a lot of church sanctuaries. The word means *a safe place*. What makes a church a sanctuary, a safe place? Let me suggest several things:

- The Word of God is spoken there.
- God is worshiped.
- Music is present.
- People seem glad to see each other.
- People wear their best.
- Handshakes and hugs take place.
- Love is spoken.
- Community is present.
- Violence is not allowed.
- Grace is offered.

When our children are babies, it is easy to identify the things they need to be safe, such as food, warmth, dry diapers, sleep, freedom from sharp edges, praise, protection from germs, and lots of touch and holding. As they grow and become more independent, we must search for the balance between protecting and providing for them and letting them go.

One of the analogies that I often use to describe this process comes from the TV show *Star Trek*. Maybe you remember this story of the starship *Enterprise* as it sailed around the universe on a voyage of discovery. When dangers approached, the captain would order that the shields be raised. This invisible barrier of some kind of atomic energy prevented bad things from getting in. Whenever the captain issued this command, he would have to call down to the engine room to make sure there was enough energy because it took lots of power to keep the shields raised. Most of the time the shields would be down, and friendly visitors and supplies could come in.

When children are born, we are the captains of their ships of discovery. We raise the shields when danger is a possibility. This takes lots of energy. At other times we let our kids sail around the universe on their own voyages of discovery, letting friendly people and nurturing supplies come in. As they grow older, they become apprentice captains of their own ships. A parent's job is to train them in how to take command.

A contemporary word for these protective shields is *boundaries*. These invisible lines of protection keep bad things out and let good things in. A home with healthy boundaries is a safe home, a sanctuary. Children are protected from invasions such as yelling and screaming, put-downs, hitting and violence, rigid self-righteous teaching and preaching, and improper sexual touch. They are being supplied with love, food, clothing, shelter, the teaching and modeling of God's love and Word, healthy touch, and respect of their personal boundaries.

Privacy

In Esther's home there was very little privacy. It was not uncommon for her parents or her older brothers or sisters to barge into the bathroom. Doors were rarely closed. Her brothers, particularly, paraded around in their underwear or in towels. Even as a young girl, Esther hated it when anyone came into the bathroom when she was taking a bath.

In a safe home, privacy is honored. This is a healthy boundary related to the privacy of one's body. The body is the temple of the Holy Spirit and should be upheld as such. Comfort levels with nudity will vary from family to family. If nakedness is treated naturally without great attention or embarrassment, it may simply be a natural part of life in a home. In Esther's home, however, there are forms of exhibitionism and voyeurism going on. Concern for her comfort or personal boundaries is absent.

At times Esther needs help from her mom or older sisters with getting dressed or, as a young girl, taking a bath. Discerning parents will sense when their children are ready to do many of these things for themselves and will allow them the freedom to do so. This may mean that some mistakes are made, like wearing the wrong colors, but allowing a child to learn from these mistakes and have the freedom of his or her own privacy is a great gift. With siblings, wise parents will enforce these safe boundaries and gently correct violations when they occur.

This respect for privacy is especially important when it comes to parents' own sexual behavior. One of the great frustrations for many couples, sexually, is the lack of privacy that goes with having children in the home. It is not an uncommon story for a child to interrupt his or her parents during sex.

Erica, age eight, couldn't sleep one night. So she wandered around and eventually walked into her parents' bedroom. There she saw her dad on top of her mom, and it looked like he might be hurting her so she said, "Dad, stop it!" Mom and Dad were obviously embarrassed but collected themselves. Erica's mom said, "Erica, Dad is not hurting me. We were having sex, just like we've talked about. This is very special, and it feels very good. I know that it might look frightening, but it is a very close time of physical touching and holding for us. It is also something that we want to do by ourselves."

Erica's dad and mom asked her to go back to her room. Then they got dressed and went to her room. They knocked and asked if it was okay to come into her room. Erica's dad said, "You know that I love your mom, and we would never hurt each other. Sex is something that married people really enjoy doing. It must look kind of strange or funny, but it is about us touching and holding each other and being really close."

Both of Erica's parents told her that sex is something that moms and dads do in private. It is a part of the special relationship just for a mom and dad to experience together. It is hard to enjoy when someone else is watching. They also explained that, in the future Erica could come and get them anytime that she really needs to, but that she needs to knock on their door before she comes in.

Children need a variety of safe boundaries as they grow up. Learning how to respect other family members' privacy is one of them. When doors are closed, people need to knock before they come in. Parents need to model this. Don't go into your child's room without knocking and asking if it is okay to come in.

Sexual Boundaries

Consider again the opening story about Elizabeth and Andrew. In addition to taking this opportunity to teach his children about gender differences and social boundaries, their father also gives them an opportunity to say if anyone else had ever asked to touch or look at their private parts. As we send our kids out into the world, we will need to occasionally investigate these possibilities without frightening them. Eighty percent of the people I work with who struggle with sexual sin were sexually abused as children. As parents you need to be aware that sexual abuse makes a child extremely vulnerable to sexual temptation and sexual problems of many kinds as they grow older.

Stories of the sexual abuse of children are rampant, as milk-carton notices remind us. Clergy, teachers, doctors, and others are being arrested and imprisoned for sexual abuse. Newspapers are full of details. Many communities are calling for mandatory reporting when sex offenders move into a neighborhood. The Internet can be a recruiting ground for naive and innocent, but curious, kids. It is crucial that we prepare our children for the dangers that are out in the world. Again, we must do this in a sensitive way so as not to frighten them unnecessarily.

As discussed in chapter 4, by this time parents should already have talked to their children about "private parts" of their bodies. This doesn't have to be complicated and is just a matter of simple explanation. In this stage, parents will need to warn their children to be careful because other people may be interested in those parts for all the wrong reasons. In part, these conversations revolve around the proverbial "Don't take candy from strangers" message. You probably already know how to talk about safety in these more general ways, but today we must recognize that "candy" is only a metaphor and comes in many different forms and wrappers.

Stuart, five years old, was an average kid who liked to play with his friends. Occasionally when both his parents had to work, Stuart would be left to occupy his time in the neighborhood. One day one of his friends had a brand-new computer game. When Stuart asked where he got it, the friend said it was from the man who lived at the end of the street and that he was really nice. Stuart decided to check this out for himself and asked his friend if he could go along with him the next time.

Several days later, Stuart stood on this man's front porch knocking on the door. When the man came to the door, he had a big smile on his face and was glad to see the boys. He had many wonderful things in his house, including all the computer equipment one could imagine, and there were always lots of fun games to share. Stuart loved going there. The man was so nice.

One day Stuart went by himself; it seemed like the logical thing to do. The man, as always, was glad to see him. They played with the computer. Then the man said to him that he had something special to show him. He clicked on several buttons, and in seconds Stuart was looking at pictures of naked men and women. Stuart was fascinated by things he had never seen before and also somewhat frightened. The man asked what he thought of all of that. Stuart didn't know what to say. Then the man asked, "Would you like to see me naked like those pictures?"

Even as I write, I'm frightened by this story, but it is typical of hundreds of stories I have heard. Current statistics indicate that one-third of all girls and one-fourth of all boys will be sexually abused between the ages of four and nine. Will Stuart be prepared to deal with something like this? The story is reflective of many things we know about sexual abuse. One of them is that the average child molester is well known to the child. The molester has gone to some length to build the victim's trust. He or she may even be a family member or a friend of the family. Stuart's parents may have even been glad that there was an adult on the block who seemed to really care about the boys.

In other situations, abusers may use emotional force to coerce children into being sexual. This can frighten children into thinking that if they ever tell anyone, they will get themselves into trouble. Sadly, many professionals, including clergy, can fall into this category. With clergy the damage is especially profound. One colleague of mine calls those clergy who perpetrate this kind of damage "slayers of the soul."

Besides adults, older children may be the most common of child abusers. Baby-sitters, neighborhood kids, even older siblings or relatives can do great damage specifically because they have access to children and are trusted members of a family or community.

If we don't have an ongoing conversation with our kids about safety and keeping certain parts of our bodies private, and if the sanctuary of our own home is not as good as it should be, it will be difficult to start a discussion by simply asking, "Has anyone tried to sexually abuse you?" They are bound to clam up. It is better, as with so many topics about sex, to have an ongoing conversation with your children about dangers.

Following are some very important messages to tell your child many different times:

- It is never okay for anyone to touch your private parts.
- It is never okay for anyone to ask you to touch their private parts.
- It is never okay for anyone to ask to see you naked or to ask you to see them naked.

- It is never okay for anyone to ask you to be sexual with someone else while they watch.
- If anyone ever asks you to do these things, leave immediately. Don't try to explain why you are leaving, just go. If you need to yell for help, do so. Go to the nearest adult you can find and ask for help.
- Anyone who tells you that you, or someone else, will get in trouble for telling is lying to you.
- If something like this ever happens, I (we) will never be mad at you.
- It is never your fault when something like this happens.
- We always want to hear about these things, and we will do our best to protect you.

Stuart ran home and immediately told his parents what had happened. After they were sure that he was physically okay and that no sexual contact had actually occurred, Stuart's dad said, "I'm so proud of you for getting out of there. You did exactly the right thing. You are a brave boy for telling us." Stuart protested, "It was really my fault for going there in the first place. I liked going there. He was such a nice man." Stuart's mom responded, "I know he seemed like a nice man, and this whole experience must be really confusing, but it is definitely not your fault. You were just doing what seemed like a nice and fun thing to do."

Both of his parents said in different ways, "It really hurts when someone you like disappoints you like this. It makes it hard to trust anyone. This is a hard lesson for you to learn, but there are people in the world whom we can trust. We hope that you trust us to take care of this and to try to keep you safe from having it happen again."

Stuart's parents reported the man. They didn't try to talk to him themselves. They knew that they were not the right kind of authority. It turned out that this was not the first time this man had been reported. Stuart's parents kept him informed of everything that was going on, repeating time and again that this wasn't his fault and that the man was going to get the kind of help he needed, even if it meant going to jail for a while. Stuart's parents also called other parents in the neighborhood to tell them of their experience so they could find out if their children had had similar experiences.

We know that child abusers pick on kids who seem vulnerable, kids who appear to be lonely, isolated, or even depressed. One of the best forms of prevention that you can provide your children is to make sure they feel loved. Here are several prescriptions:

- Touch them daily.
- Hug them.
- Praise them.
- Find meaningful activities to occupy their minds.
- Help them to find safe social activities.

Wise parents will also be watchful for signs that their child is being abused by people outside the home. Here are some indicators and symptoms to watch for:

- a change in mood from a happy child to one who seems moody or depressed
- fear of certain people or places
- increasing amounts of time spent in isolation
- behavior that imitates sexual acts
- preoccupation with sexual innuendo, jokes, or talk
- preoccupation with going to the bathroom, taking baths, or dressing
- itching, particularly in genital areas
- vaginal discharge
- bruises

Many of these could be symptoms of other kinds of problems or abuse. It is always preventive to err on the side of investigation conducted in a gentle, caring, understanding, and thoughtful way that doesn't continue the invasion.

Peter, age six, was being sexually abused by an older teenage boy in the neighborhood. He seemed afraid of going outside, and he avoided any possibility of seeing this boy. He was moody. The quality of his schoolwork was declining. Peter seemed much more obsessed with the privacy of his own room.

His father came into his room one night and said, "Peter, I'm really worried about you. You seem sad a lot. You also seem generally afraid. Your schoolwork is slipping. Please know that I am not mad at you in any way, but I wonder what is going on. Nothing that you are doing could ever stop me or Mom from loving you. We are here to love and protect you. If someone is doing something wrong or painful to you, it is not your fault. We want to know so that we can do something about it. It may be frightening to even think about talking about these things, but you need to know that we love you and will help you."

Peter may need to get some specialized help to work through his experience, but his father has done the right thing. His actions and words are not invasive. It is his job to protect his son.

Catch your breath. This is a lot of work and you may find that, given your own background, you are not good at handling these issues. Find help from adults, teachers, pastors, and others whom you trust. Protecting your child's sexual boundaries is the hard, but crucial, work of parenting.

HEALTHY SEXUALITY DURING EARLY CHILDHOOD: SPIRITUAL DIMENSION

Kids will also be learning what is morally right and wrong during this stage. This is the beginning of discovering their own God-given conscience and developing it, which is also vitally important during this stage.

Conscience is developed socially and culturally by the shifting norms and values of our time. A child's sense of moral value at these early ages may simply be one of conformity. He or she will do what others are doing. Parents will need to monitor what their children are learning about morality in general and certainly about sex in particular. Even seemingly innocuous television shows or magazine covers will be sending messages.

Suzie, age eight, liked going to the grocery store with her mom. Her mom always bought her a treat, and they had fun together. Suzie was learning to read more and more things. As they checked out one particular day, Suzie was looking at the magazine covers as her mom paid the cashier. Her eyes focused on one particular issue of a popular women's magazine. The lead article said, "How to Have an Affair Without Hurting Your Husband." In the car on the way home, Suzie asked her mom, "What's an affair?"

This is actually a relatively tame article compared to some I've seen recently. It would not be uncommon to hear questions these days about particular sexual practices, orgasm, infidelity, or how to be more sexually attractive. While parents may need to provide technical information about these things, the fact that these kind of images and words are in "normal" places tends to "normalize" the activities to which they refer, especially in young minds.

Suzie's parents had already talked to her about sex, so Suzie's mom didn't have to start responding to her daughter's question from scratch. "An affair usually is when two people who are not married to each other have sex," she explained. "Sometimes this can mean that they have sex one time, or it can mean that they have sex regularly. God teaches us in his commandments that this is adultery and is sinful. It always hurts those involved in some way. That magazine is not right, and that is one of the reasons why Dad and I don't buy them and will always encourage you not to read them. This may be hard for you because I imagine many of your other friends will be having that kind of magazine around. I hope that you will always feel free to come to Dad or me and talk about any questions you have about what you read."

Jesus taught us that we live in the world but should not be of the world. This is not an easy assignment for children or their parents. A child will be learning a set of messages at home and at church that may not be affirmed by other sources of information in their world. It is critical, especially with sex, that parents talk to children often about these confusing messages. As Christians we should understand that there is a difference between a spiritual understanding and a social awareness of what is right and wrong. We are responsible to teach our children not only the social "rules" that will keep them "out of trouble," but also the precious truths of Scripture that will protect them and fill them with true wisdom. "Your statutes are my delight; they are my counselors" (Psalm 119:24). In this stage of development, parents must do everything they can to instruct children in God's law.

We live in a confusing time. Many people, even Christians, have become desensitized to the sexual stimuli that surround us. If you are very brave, carry a notebook with you for a day and write down every sexual image, message, or stimulus that you encounter in your routine day. Then imagine what it might be like for your children even in their slightly more protected world. We live in a time when so many of our respected leaders, including clergy, have fallen sexually. This is not to mention the sexual sinfulness of many of our revered entertainers and sports heroes. Last night at the drugstore I saw a five-year-old looking at the picture of a naked woman on the back of a popular magazine. Yesterday, I got a call from a mother who asked, "How do I talk to my seven-year-old son about the fact that the president of the United States had sex in the Oval Office?" I have also sat in groups of parents who were struggling with how to talk to their children about the fact that the pastor of their church had sex with a number of the boys in the youth group.

The deceptions of Satan are legion. In Genesis 3:2-4 we see the first one:

> The woman said to the serpent, "We may eat fruit from the trees in the garden, but God did say, 'You must not eat fruit from the tree that is in the middle of the garden, and you must not touch it, or you will die.'"
>
> "You will not surely die," the serpent said to the woman.

The lie is that we won't "die" if we sin. Teaching our children that this is a lie will be an essential ingredient of our moral instruction to them about anything including sexuality. Sexual sin can bring death to the possibility of true intimacy with a spouse. Sexual sin may even bring physical death through sexually transmitted disease. It is a lie that sexual sin is no big deal, that everyone is doing it.

The challenge is how to teach the truth to our kids and still allow them the freedom to make their own mistakes. My basic answer is that we teach them the truth, and then we practice what we preach. If we make mistakes, we admit them and try to do better. Punishing our kids for their mistakes is usually not the best way to help them develop a healthy conscience, one that is sensitive to the loving Spirit of God who must ultimately guide them in life. Some people who grow up with harsh judgment, criticism, and/or physical punishment as the tools for teaching right and wrong may become "riddled" with conscience. People who grow up in this kind of environment may become so legalistic and rigid that they can hardly function. They become afraid of breaking the law because of the harsh ways in which they learned it.

As parents we must be careful about how we teach God's law. We don't want kids thinking only that God is harsh and vengeful. Discipline that includes phrases like "Jesus will hate you for that" or "God will punish you for that" may teach kids the message that "Jesus hates me, this I know, for my parents tell me so." Jesus frequently confronted the rather paranoid Pharisees and teachers of the law who were continually worried that he was violating some rule. Jesus reminded them in Matthew 5:17 that he didn't come to abolish the Law, but to fulfill it.

Listen to the rest of the conversation that Suzie's mom had with her.

"When God tells us not to have affairs, he is not trying prevent us from having fun. He is trying to tell us that being faithful to our husband or wife is the highest form of love that two people can have. If they were to be sexual with others, that would hurt both of them very much and violate that kind of love. Your dad and I try to love each other in this way. God wants us to be faithful to each other. This is the only way that we can really know the best kind of love.

"I can tell you that I love your dad so much that I would never hurt him by hav-

ing an affair. This kind of love is such a special feeling and is something that will be hard for you to fully understand until you meet that man whom you love so much that you will want to spend your whole life with him."

As parents we are going to have to continually point out to our kids the lies that are prevalent in our culture, especially in music, TV, movies, and magazines. The task of talking to your children about sex is a lifetime journey of instruction, example, and practice at how to discern the truth and live according to it in love.

HEALTHY SEXUALITY CHECKLIST

Now let's review our model of healthy sexuality and look at the learning objectives of this age group.

Physical. Children in this age span will be naturally curious and inquisitive. Self-touching and sex play are common during this stage and should be responded to with wisdom and understanding. Children in this age span will understand the basic mechanics of genital sexuality. They will also be aware of the basic nature of pregnancy and the process of birth and delivery. Special attention will be given to helping them understand the differences between males and females.

Emotional. Children will learn how to talk about their emotions. They will be affirmed when they are honest about how they feel and encouraged to be open about their thoughts. Parents will model appropriate ways to express anger, sadness, and loneliness. Parents will be aware if a child is alone too often or using behaviors to "medicate" his or her feelings.

Relational. Parents will encourage their children to have appropriate friendships and allow them to play. Special attention will be given to modeling healthy social interaction between males and females. Children will learn accepted social boundaries and interact appropriately.

Personal. Parents will provide safety within the family and make sure their home is a sanctuary. Privacy will be respected, and personal and sexual wounds will be prevented. Instruction will be given to children about personal boundaries and how to avoid abusive situations. Parents will be careful to monitor any symptoms of possible sexual abuse.

Spiritual. Children will be forming a personal conscience and learning to discern what is morally right and wrong. Parents will begin to teach the basic foundation of God's law, both in its specific rules and in its spirit. Children will come to understand that people of faith will often be in conflict with the culture and that being children of God sometimes may require standing alone or being different.

Remember that development varies and that some kids grow faster physically, emotionally, and spiritually than others. You may find that you already need to address with your eight- or nine-year-olds some of the issues we cover in the next chapter. Let's turn now to the ten-to-fourteen age group, one of the most tumultuous times for our children in terms of their developing sexuality.

CHAPTER SIX

Puberty

(A G E   1 0 – 1 4)

Bob, age thirteen, stood in the locker room after gym class. Some of the boys were show-
ering; others were just getting dressed. He was trying to decide which of these two things
to do himself. He didn't want to stink up his next class, but he felt embarrassed about
taking a shower with the other boys. Some of them seemed so much bigger and more
developed than he was. They had hair in certain places he didn't yet. He felt pretty inad-
equate and wondered if he would get teased. Another part of him just felt plain awk-
ward about being naked in a public place. The gym teacher came up and said, "Bob,
what are you waiting for? Either get dressed and get out of here or hit the showers."

YOUR CHILD'S BASIC DEVELOPMENTAL TASKS

One of the biggest changes kids in this age group face is the wide range of
physical development that will occur. The instigator of these changes is the
pituitary gland at the base of the brain. It is programmed to release hormones and start various physical activities at certain points of development.
The whole process is called puberty. Some of you may have an emotional
reaction at the mention of the word because it brings back many memories
of being different and awkward.

Both boys and girls will experience physical changes of size, hair growth, and bodily function during this time. Girls will start menstruating. Boys may experience their first nocturnal emission. A majority of boys and some girls will have learned how to masturbate. Feelings of attraction for the opposite sex may surprise them because of earlier dislikes. This is also the stage when homosexual feelings may occur for some and be very confusing. Fantasies of sexual activity may take hold. For boys, fantasy will be more visual; for girls, relational.

This is the stage in which we traditionally think sexual information should be presented. By this time, however, we should have already communicated quite a bit about sex and its biological particulars to our kids. If they haven't heard it from us, they will already know about sex from school, friends, or some channel of our culture. If children aren't prepared for the massive physical and emotional changes that will take place in them, they will be surprised and confused by them.

The latest studies suggest that the average age of first intercourse for boys is seventeen and for girls, sixteen. If this is the average, then some in this earlier stage will certainly be experimenting with various levels of sexual contact. If a child has been sexually or physically abused in earlier stages, this is also the stage in which his or her sexual activity will begin to reflect in some way the nature of that abuse.

In this stage of childhood, these are the primary developmental tasks kids need to accomplish in order to continue developing healthy sexuality:

- knowing how their own body works and how it is changing and developing
- understanding sex, procreation, and childbirth
- being able to understand and communicate feelings
- knowing what sexual behaviors might be used to block or change negative feelings
- knowing what sexual behaviors might be used as substitutes for love and nurture

- having healthy and mutual relationships with males and females
- knowing that they are accepted for who they really are
- feeling attractive and not being frightened by the thought of sex
- being oriented to the opposite sex
- maturing spiritually without losing childlike faith
- being able to participate in a Christian community and knowing that they belong; finding trusted authorities to model faith to them

YOUR PRIMARY PARENTING TASKS

If you're a woman, did you experience your first menstrual cycle with little or no preparation? If you're a man, did you experience your first "wet dream" without anyone telling you it could happen? What do you remember about your own sexual feelings during this stage? Use the energy of these memories to motivate you to talk to your kids. All of these questions raise topics that parents must not only be willing to discuss, but initiate conversations about.

Recall from your own experience that this is one of those phases of life that is truly transitional. A girl becomes a woman, and a boy becomes a man—at least physically, if not emotionally and spiritually. In modern American culture, this transition is too often dreaded or feared by parents, when in fact it should be celebrated. In many other times of human history and in other cultures, people have done a better job of celebrating childhood rites of passage. Primitive peoples perform various initiation rites that signify to others that a child has completed one stage of development and is entering another. A boy is now a man of the tribe, a hunter, a provider. A girl is now a woman capable of being married and of bearing children. Jewish culture celebrates this transition spiritually when they bar mitzvah a boy and bat mitzvah a girl. Now they are ready to study Scripture with the men or women and be an adult in the eyes of the temple.

How are you honoring this "coming of age" in your child's life? How will you celebrate it with your child? I suggest that you create some ritual in your family that signifies this change. Find a strategy that is meaningful to you. Take your child out to dinner, have a party, give him or her something that symbolizes growing up. Let your children know that you recognize their growth and development.

This doesn't mean teasing them about their changing bodies or their new romantic interests. Make sure that whatever you do honors your child. A woman once told me that at a family gathering, her father announced to the entire extended family that she had started menstruating and was now a woman. She, of course, was mortified. We need to stay away from anything that would embarrass our children. We therefore need to confer with them about what would be meaningful to them.

Don't make the mistake of thinking that you can take them out, have a single conversation about being an adult and about sexuality, and be done with your responsibility in this area. Remember that, whatever you do, you will have a series of conversations. Perhaps you can schedule a series of outings during which you discuss the topics covered in this chapter. Your tasks during this complex stage include:

- making sure your children have a full understanding about sex, the process of conception, and childbirth
- affirming them physically, emotionally, and spiritually
- touching them in nonsexual ways
- providing them correct, biblical moral boundaries while not overreacting to the mistakes associated with their experimentation
- being aware of the symptoms of problem sexual behaviors and getting help if needed
- encouraging them to have healthy friendships
- celebrating with them their transition into adulthood
- providing them with opportunities to be with trusted Christian mentors who will also be models

HEALTHY SEXUALITY DURING PUBERTY: PHYSICAL DIMENSION

Awkwardness

For some children, the hormonal changes that signal the start of puberty will begin at ages eight to nine. For some, puberty will start as late as seventeen or eighteen. For most, however, it will begin between ten and fourteen years of age. Go to any middle school or junior high today, and you will see a picture of diversity. Some kids will still look very much like children. Others will be as big or bigger than you. Some boys will have large muscles and already be shaving. Their voices will be deep and rich. Some girls will have developed the roundness of their bodies including wider hips and larger breasts. Most, whatever their place in the wide range of normal development, will be thinking that they are totally different and weird. Studies suggest that 80 percent of adolescents are terribly self-conscious about their appearance and don't like how they look during these years.

Martha, age thirteen, was very petite. Most people thought she was really cute. She hadn't grown as fast, however, as some of the girls around her and she felt too small. This was bad enough, but most of the girls had started wearing bras because they needed them. Martha's mom had taken her out to get some, but one day in school several of the boys teased her, saying, "What do you need that for?"

Martha was mortified and was obviously withdrawn when she came home. Martha's mother had been sensitive to this possibility and suspected what was going on. She went into Martha's room and asked her if she could talk. Martha started crying. After just holding her for a while, her mom asked her what it was about. Martha cried, "All the boys hate me!"

After the day's events had been clarified, Martha's mom said, "Honey, that must have really hurt. Those boys were insensitive and wrong in what they said. You're at that age when even some of your friends will tease each other about their bodies. You are all changing at different rates. One of the ways people cover their own self-

consciousness about their bodies is to tease others about theirs. It's not right, but it happens.

"I want you to know that I think you are a beautiful girl, and God is not yet finished with your figure. Let me show you something." At that point, Martha's mom got out some pictures of herself when she was thirteen. She looked a lot like Martha in every way. As an adult, Martha's mom had a very attractive figure, and even though Martha had seen these pictures before, she finally focused on how her mom had changed as she grew up. Her mom went on to tell her that many boys had teased her, too, and that it was painful. "When my breasts finally got bigger, I was so relieved. I used to pray every night that they would grow, but God has built a different plan into all bodies. It's hard right now to accept this, but whatever your figure is like one day, both Dad and I are praying that you will find a man who loves you for your spirit. If you find such a man, the size of any part of your body will be beautiful to him."

During puberty, your children will need constant reassurance that they are physically attractive. They will need you to comfort them in their feelings of being different, ugly, and awkward. They may act as if they don't want to be touched, but they still need hugs or pats on the shoulder. Young adolescents are naturally good at trying to ease their own feelings of inadequacy by teasing or making fun of others. Do not participate in this teasing, but be ready to offer appropriate affirmations.

Cynthia was feeling really proud that her mom had taken her to buy her first bra, but she felt nervous and awkward about wearing it. What would the boys think? What would her dad think? Cynthia's dad felt awkward too. When he first saw her wearing it he said, "What's this?" With that, he reached around her, pulled on the back of her bra, and snapped it. "Wow, the boys are going to be all over you now."

This is one of those examples of a father regressing to his own adolescent feelings of uneasiness. He didn't know what to do in response to this new stage in Cynthia's life or how to reassure his daughter in a positive and healthy way. A mature father might simply say, "I'm really proud of you. You're growing up into a beautiful woman."

David had started growing some facial hair but not much. He took great pride in getting out his dad's razor and shaving. One day his mom saw him doing this, came into the bathroom, felt his cheek, and said, "You don't really need to worry about this peach fuzz."

This comment was thoughtless but was not intended to be malicious. Perhaps David's mom just didn't want him to grow up too fast. She failed to realize how important this activity was to her growing son. She might have simply said, "Wow, you're really starting to become a man."

Preparing to Procreate

God's age-old design of creation is preparing children at this time for their reproductive roles. Greater amounts of the chemical hormone testosterone begins to circulate in boys, often felt as the "raging hormone" because of the sudden intensity of sexual feeling. The vestige of a protective layer of hair all over the body begins to appear. Muscles will grow, a boy's penis will get larger, and his testicles will further develop so as to equip him for his role in the planting of human "seeds." Occasionally, boys will ejaculate at night. Sexual arousal is a nocturnal experience for all men. In this stage, with no other sexual outlet, the body will take over and produce an occasional orgasm, sometimes called a "wet dream." These are normal and not about any out-of-control sexual dreams.

Estrogen is the hormonal agent in girls' bodies. As estrogen levels increase, girls will develop wider hips for childbirth and larger breasts for nursing. The ovaries and uterus will start going through regular monthly cycles of receptivity to the male's seed.

Everything about the female's physical features—her hair, her feet, her breasts, her legs, her buttocks—will begin to be wildly attractive to the male. The male's strength, expressed in his muscles, his strong voice, and his eyes, will be attractive to the female. She will develop strong biological and sexual reactions in her brain to receive the male's seed and produce children. Some sociologists and anthropologists teach that, biologically, we are programmed to pair off at these ages and to begin to reproduce the species. In this sense, they would say, we have been taught to delay gratification. Many adolescents and teenagers are, naturally, tempted not to wait.

Christians know that we are called to a higher spiritual connection between a husband and wife. We believe it is important to delay our biological sexual urges for a higher purpose, not just because of some modern-day cultural development. Part of a parent's job is to reassure their children that their biological drives are normal and nothing to be afraid of.

You will need to have many conversations with your children about the physical developments in their bodies during puberty. Although you will have already talked to them about the basic biology of human sexuality and reproduction, you will need to have a series of conversations during this time that may seem repetitive. One of the reasons for this is to reinforce correct information. Your children will be encountering lots of misinformation from their friends and from the culture. If your kids are in public or private schools, don't assume that they are getting all the instruction they need. Familiarize yourself with school's sex-education curriculum so that you can fill in any gaps. It is always better to have this information reinforced rather than ignored by parents. Addressing the topic within the home also gives your children opportunities to ask any specific questions they may have.

Boys and girls will obviously need to hear information that is specific to their development, about erections and nocturnal emissions or about breast development and menstruation. They will also need to learn about developmental changes in the opposite sex.

I remember a time when I was twelve that one of my female friends didn't want to go swimming with the group. She didn't say why. She'd always liked swimming. I didn't know about the possible embarrassment of menstruation. My mother said to me, "Leave her alone." I didn't know what she was talking about. It would have been a great time for my parents to explain things to me. As it was, girls continued to be a great mystery.

I didn't have basic information about them and was really in the dark. I didn't know how to talk to them. I had no way of trying to understand them. More importantly, I was left vulnerable to what other influences of culture, like pornography, taught me about women. Such ignorance can fuel a young adolescent's curiosity and experimentation. In a quest to find out what he doesn't know, he may do inappropriate things, including sexual ones, to find out more.

Most of all, ignorance produces feelings of loneliness and isolation. In the face of that, many kids choose substitutes for intimacy that are not healthy. The fact that a young person has adequate knowledge suggests that someone loved him or her enough to share this information. The presence of love in his or her life is a part of healthy sexual development in obvious ways. If kids have basic information about what is going on with their own bodies and with each other during this stage, they will be less frightened and embarrassed, less likely to tease each other, less likely to experiment in search of answers, and less likely to turn to those who may teach them the wrong answers.

HEALTHY SEXUALITY DURING PUBERTY: EMOTIONAL DIMENSION

The same physical hormones that prepare a child for sexual development may also create some havoc in the brain emotionally. For some there will be great swings of emotions from high to low. Adolescents may be angry and volatile for no apparent reason. At other times they may be feel overwhelmingly sad and cry without knowing why.

Hormonal surges will vary genetically from child to child and may be expressed differently in girls than in boys. Many women now know about the nature of cyclical monthly emotions. Oftentimes right before a period starts, there will be feelings of depression, anger, and irritability. As you know, this has come to be called premenstrual syndrome (PMS) and is usually medically treatable.

Because of the many "strange" things going on in a child's body during this stage, he or she may struggle with feelings of shame or embarrassment. Otherwise outgoing children may now seem shy and withdrawn. New sexual feelings, if not explained, may lead them to think that they are "bad" or perverted. Humor and criticism of others may be a cover for their feelings of shame.

Because of the close connection between physical and emotional development during this stage, parents will need to continue closely monitoring how their child is coping with feeling different, embarrassed, or shameful. What are they doing to feel like they fit in? Are they processing their conflicting emotions or covering them up with various behaviors that could stunt their emotional growth? As we discussed in the previous chapter, healthy development in the emotional dimension involves dealing honestly with feelings rather than repressing or projecting them. During puberty, it is especially critical to help children make healthy connections between their emotions and their sexuality. If emotional development lags behind sexual development, sexual problems can easily develop.

Two potential problem areas are very common in this stage and may influence your child's sexual development if not addressed effectively.

Masturbation

Peter, age thirteen, discovered touching himself genitally when he was a small boy. It felt pleasurable, and he really didn't think anything about it. As he grew older, he found himself doing it more and more. One day, when he was eleven, a strange thing happened. He ejaculated. It surprised him, and he wondered if something was wrong. No one had ever talked to him about this kind of thing happening. Even though he was worried, nothing else bad seemed to happen and so the next day he tried it again. This continued. At first he didn't really need to think about anything to experience it.

More and more, as he grew older, he found that he would need to think about some sexual fantasy in order to have an orgasm. Gradually, the sexual fantasies got more elaborate. Peter found that looking at pornography helped him to fantasize more creatively, which led to an even more intense sexual high during masturbation.

As we discussed in chapter 5, masturbation is the act of self-stimulating one's genital area and is a normal part of development as one discovers one's own body. There is no specific biblical injunction against masturbation, and we should not automatically lump it in with a list of sexual perversions or sexual sins. I believe that the answer to whether or not masturbation is normal during this stage of childhood is more complex because of the emotional and spiritual issues that may be connected to it.

In the Sermon on the Mount Jesus said these familiar words: "You have heard that it was said, 'Do not commit adultery.' But I tell you that anyone who looks at a woman lustfully has already committed adultery with her in his heart" (Matthew 5:27-28). Jesus was not talking about masturbation specifically but about the secret thoughts a person might have about being sexual with others. It seems clear that Jesus was condemning the heart attitude that results in obsessively lusting after a person who is not one's spouse.

It is normal to be attracted to members of the opposite sex, and given the nature of our current culture, it would be almost impossible to go through a day without some sort of sexual stimulation. Some of this stimulation may lead to sexual thoughts. I don't think that passing sexual thoughts are what Jesus was referring to in the verse above; rather, I believe he was talking about sinful lust. Lust is obsessive thinking or fantasizing about someone that goes way beyond simple thoughts. Like so many things, we should be careful to remember that sexual fantasy is not good or bad in a black-and-white sense. Sexual fantasy is sinful if it causes a person to fantasize lustfully about sex outside the boundary of marriage.

When very young children masturbate, sexual lust is obviously not an issue. As kids get older, however, and the physical pleasure they experience during masturbation becomes overtly sexual, they are more likely to fantasize about remembered or imagined sexual experience. It may be that the act of masturbation is not inherently sinful; it really depends on what a person fantasizes about while stimulating himself. This would make it rather difficult to imagine that masturbation for an adolescent is a healthy practice if it is a regular habit accompanied by fantasizing about sexual experience outside of marriage. So while we should not judge this age group for experimenting with masturbation as a way of understanding and exploring their bodies, we must look to the deeper question of the fantasies behind its practice. In my illustration with Peter, note that his habit grew, and it came to include more elaborate fantasies and eventually even pornography. This clearly is leading him in a dangerous direction.

What is the purpose of any kind of fantasy? One possible purpose is that it creates an escape, a diversion from one's own reality. A person can literally imagine any possible scenario, any prospective partner, any possible sexual practice. If a person's reality is rather lonely, fantasy offers an escape. If a person's marriage is not so good, a better partner can be imagined. If sex in a relationship is not so good, better sex can be imagined.

Obsessive fantasizing and masturbation reflect on the emotional health of an adolescent. These activities may, and usually do, indicate that the child is lonely or frustrated with friendships, family, or life in general. Fantasy can create elaborate escapes from the reality of one's own loneliness. If the basic nature of this loneliness is not addressed, coping mechanisms will continue to be constructed and healthy emotional development will be thwarted. Fantasizing about the perfect lover in order to feel less lonely is never the real answer and always leads to further dissatisfaction. Sexual fantasy, masturbation, or any other kind of sexual activity is not the answer to legitimate emotional needs.

Don't get freaked out if you discover that your young adolescent is masturbating. Work, however, to get to the bottom of the issue. Talk to him or her. Find out what your child is feeling. Help him or her to understand that sexual fantasy is never a real solution to loneliness or emotional problems.

Peter's mom accidentally walked in on him one day when he was masturbating. She didn't quite know what to say, but she was wise enough not to make a big deal about it then. Later, Peter's mom and dad had the following talk with him over dinner.

"Son, the last thing that we want to do is embarrass you by talking to you about masturbation," Peter's dad said. "It is a very common practice for boys your age to masturbate. I have certainly done it. I did it when I was your age. I remember how shameful I sometimes felt while at the same time it felt so good. In many ways this is a form of discovering your body and how it works. I remember trying to explain to you what an orgasm was. Now, in a way, you know. It is also really normal to be attracted to girls and to have sexual thoughts about them. I'm glad that you're becoming a man and having these kind of thoughts."

Peter's mom added, "I also would like you to know that what you are doing is totally normal. I certainly don't think any less of you or love you less because you've done this. I would still say that having an orgasm by yourself is really different from how it will feel with your future wife. There is so much more to the experience when you combine it with the intimacy of marriage."

Peter's parents went on to tell him about the relationship between fantasy and masturbation and the dangers of it becoming too frequent for all the wrong reasons. They told him that when Jesus taught about the sin of lusting, he was also pointing to the very special relationship that should exist between a man and a woman. Our faith teaches us that there are things we choose to deny ourselves so that we can experience higher relationships. This is not always easy, but many things in life aren't.

Finally, they said, "If you're ever lonely or angry and feel bad about something in your life, we hope that you'll let us know so that we can help you find real solutions to those problems. Never be afraid to talk to us about anything."

Pornography

Stan, age ten, came home one day and told his dad that some of the guys at school had been passing around a magazine that depicted the most private parts of naked women. He told his dad that he had looked at it, and he felt really bad.

Looking at depictions of naked people is not inherently evil. Whether or not such depictions are pornographic depends on how they are portrayed and how they are perceived. When I refer to pornography, I am talking about the vast volume of material out there that would stimulate most people in a sexually immoral way. Some of the responsibility for labeling something as pornographic, however, belongs to the beholder. Consider, for example, the classic statue of King David sculpted by Michelangelo, on display in Florence, Italy. David is naked, and his penis is as well defined as only the great master sculptor could make it. If this visual stimulus excites a sexual drive that is immoral, would we say that this statue is pornographic? At least part of that responsibility belongs to those looking at it.

However, great works of art are not the focus of concern for most parents. Today's proliferation of magazines, videos, and Web sites depict not only naked men and women, but sexual intercourse, sex with children, sex with animals, sadomasochistic or violent sex, homosexual sex, and sex with multiple partners. Someone showed me a "menu" of more than one hundred different sexual activities that were portrayed on just one foreign Web site. Some of these were so bizarre that I hope they are beyond your imagination. More than two thousand new pornographic videos are produced each week. Popularly accepted magazines have more and more sexual images and articles in them. Most of all, the Internet now provides pornography so easily that your average grade-schooler can access it without any difficulty.

If you want to protect your children from this onslaught of sexually graphic images, then you had better be prepared both to talk to them about why pornography is dangerous and to take action to prohibit their access to it. Much of what was covered in the section on masturbation and fantasy applies here. Looking at pictures and lusting after sex partners outside the bounds of marriage is hardly in keeping with biblical mandates, and it certainly does not contribute to healthy emotional development as it relates to sexuality and future intimacy with a spouse. Looking at or reading pornography may also excite the brain chemistry, resulting in an addiction that leads the brain to demand more and more.

Whether we are consciously aware of it or not, pornography sends strong messages to the mind and spirit as well as the body. As you consider having a conversation with your child about pornography, let's examine some of the myths that pornography teaches.

Everyone is having sex. The sheer volume of what's out there would lead you to believe that sex is everywhere. Pornography never suggests that any moral or spiritual choice is involved. It is simply assumed that a person should find as much sex as possible and that such promiscuity is not something that should ever bother your conscience or anyone else's. One of the problems with this myth is that you can feel rather left out if you aren't having lots of sex.

Sex is for recreation. This myth assumes that even if two people aren't friends, or don't have a relationship of any kind, sex would be a fun thing to do. Pornography is full of total strangers who have supposedly chance encounters. Since their biological drives are running the show, why not just have sex? What's the big deal?

The people who are portrayed are really enjoying it. In most pornography, sex always seems wildly fulfilling. No one ever complains or struggles with a decision, and their faces are always smiling if not rapturous. This myth suggests that all people really enjoy sex, regardless of the nature of it or the people with whom they are having it.

Sex is always exciting. In pornography, everyone usually has an orgasm. Everyone is fulfilled; no one is disappointed. Sex is an adventure, another mountain to climb, another partner to discover.

Abusive sex is pleasurable. Some pornographic images portray situations in which people appear to enjoy being abused, even violently, during sexual activity. This myth teaches that even when you get hurt, sex is exciting and enjoyable.

It is okay to trick people into having sex. An old theme of pornography is that one person may have to surprise or trick the other into being sexual. Once sex begins, however, the one who has been tricked enjoys the experience. This myth fuels the phenomenon of date rape. If you believe this myth, you will think that even if your partner at first says no, she will eventually like what you're doing.

The more partners you have, the better the experience. Much pornography displays many people having sex at the same time. It is very common for two men to be with one woman or two women to be with one man. Beyond that, the more the merrier as far as pornography is concerned.

The more variety you have, the greater the experience. Another common myth is that one person should educate another, more naive person about new sexual techniques or activities. The naive person always enjoys the new experience, the assumption being that the more different kinds of sex you have, the more fun it will be.

People who "love" each other are entitled to have sex even if they aren't married. Pornography equates love and sex. Even if you are just biologically attracted to someone, you should have sex with them. Certainly if you "love" them, then it is your right to be sexual.

Married people enjoy having their partners be with someone else. A lot of pornography shows how exciting it is when your spouse is sexual with another person. The suggestion is that it will "spice up" a relationship to have this kind of variety. Some magazines show pictures that men have taken of their wives or vice versa, and videos now show "home movies" that couples have taken of themselves.

You are a prude if you don't like lots of sex. Some pornography portrays the "nerd"—someone whose religious or moral beliefs make him "priggish" about sex. He will be seduced into being sexual and will always wind up liking it. The myth is that the person has been liberated out of his repressive and "unhealthy" emotional state.

I married the wrong person. If one's spouse is not as attractive or sexually willing or exciting as the people portrayed in pornography, then we can be tempted to think, "I made a mistake. I need to find a person who loves lots of sex, all kinds of sex, all the time." The fact is, people do things in pornography that most spouses would find uncomfortable or repulsive.

These are some of the messages that your kids will be taking into their spirit if they get involved with pornographic magazines, videos, or Web sites. As parents, your task involves conveying one central message: "All these things are lies. They are myths. Don't believe them even if the rest of the world seems to."

Here is what Stan's dad said to him when Stan admitted he'd looked at the pornographic magazine with his friends.

"I'm really glad that you came to me with this, Son. Let me tell you first that I don't think you were bad for wanting to look at it. At your age it's very natural to want to look at naked women. You are curious about what they look like, and you will feel very powerful feelings of sexual excitement when you do. That is normal. God is preparing your body for the time when you will be married and want to have children. Powerful chemicals in your body called hormones will cause you to feel this way. If you haven't noticed already, you probably will soon realize that looking at these kind of pictures may cause you to have an erection. You remember that we have already talked about that. Another thing we have talked about is having fantasies. All of this may tempt you to want to have an orgasm. Again, this is a normal feeling.

"When I was your age, I got really involved in looking at the kind of magazines you looked at today. I kept a stack of them in the garage for years and would look at them when I thought that Grandma and Grandpa weren't looking. This led to many experiences of masturbating and feeling really frustrated, and I found myself becoming

more and more drawn to these images, even when I was an adult. It took me a long time and lots of help from God to get over this problem. Even though I hadn't met your mom yet, when I looked at those pictures, it really wasn't fair to her because of the many incorrect messages that pornography taught me about sex. After we did get married, I had unrealistic and unfair expectations of her and of what sex should be like. I've had to apologize to her about that.

"You see, pornography teaches many things about sex that simply are wrong. They are not about God's plan for how he wants us to enjoy sex with a wife. Once you get started looking at pornography, you may only want more; it will never be enough. You'll encounter lots of pressure out there to look at pornography and lots of teasing if you don't want to. You may feel left out if you say no."

In later conversations Stan's dad continued to remind him of the false messages that pornography delivers and to encourage him to talk about his feelings and temptations. You may be tempted to think that telling Stan all of these things will make him more susceptible to looking at pornography. My experience is that the opposite is true. Without question, exposing children to pornography will make them more likely look at it again, but talking to them about it, even sharing one's own story about it, takes the mystery away. Satan works on the naturally curious mind, tempting it to find out what it knows nothing about.

Stan's dad didn't try to teach his son everything there was to know about the dangers of pornography all by himself. He told his wife what Stan had experienced, and she also took part in talking to Stan about it. One afternoon that same week, Stan's mom took him out for ice cream and talked with him.

"Dad told me that he had shared with you about pornography. First of all, let me say that I, too, think this is very normal for you to want to look at it. You are still my wonderful son, even if you've looked at it or if you will look at it again. But I want to share some things with you now from my heart. I'd even like to think that I'm speaking for the girl who will one day be your wife.

"I hate pornography. It is abusive to women. The women in those magazines are prisoners to their need for attention from men and maybe even from other women. Pornography exploits their bodies. It leads men, even boys like you, to think that women are only to be sought after for their bodies and the pleasure they can give men. Your dad was honest with you about how he used to have a problem with pornography. When he compared me and our sexual relationship to what those magazines taught him to expect, it really hurt me. I thought that I wasn't good enough for him, that I wasn't attractive, that he didn't love me. Today I know that he does love me, and he has stopped looking at all that stuff.

"It's important for you to understand that women don't really want men to like them just for their bodies. Some women think that their bodies are the only way they will get attention. In your life many girls will try to get you to like them because they are attractive or sexy. Even when they do that, they are doing what they've learned, and it's a mistake. In the Garden of Eden when God created the first woman, Eve, he said that she was to be a companion to Adam. Girls really want you to be their friend. They will want you to like them for their spirit and their mind.

"God wants you to be attracted to girls physically, but there is so much more to a good relationship than that. Pornography will teach you all the wrong messages about women and sex, about what they like, how they act, what they will want from you and will do for you. Believe me, your dad and I are friends first. Sex is an important part of our relationship, otherwise you wouldn't be here, but we share so much more than that. Would you be willing to honor your future wife by not filling your mind with the wrong ideas about what she should look like or do?

"Son, you are such a terrific boy, I love you so much. Someday you will be a wonderful husband. I've told you many times, and I'll tell you again now: If you ever have any questions about how I think or feel, please ask."

What a gift it is for a mother to talk to her son in this way. She shared her anger about the damage done by pornography, but she was not angry with her son. She was loving and honest. She shared her own pain. She told the truth. She challenged her son. She affirmed him. She left the door open for future conversations. Stan is now less likely to get into trouble with pornography as he develops emotionally and sexually. Conversations like this with both his parents will help prepare him to be the kind of husband God wants him to be.

HEALTHY SEXUALITY DURING PUBERTY: RELATIONAL DIMENSION

Personal Identity

The emotional feelings of inadequacy about their bodies and who they are as independent individuals will lead adolescents to want to fit in. The dangerous agent here, as you know, is that age-old demon called "peer pressure." Children will be wondering if they are wearing the right clothes, if they come from families that have enough money, or if they are smart enough.

Adolescents will want to fit in with certain groups. We may be exasperated by the type of kids they choose to be with. They may also form dramatic friendships in which they swear their undying affection and loyalty one week, only to be mad at each other the next. They may also experience intense feelings of physical and emotional attraction to the opposite sex. Adolescents may date or "go together." I am still trying to figure out from my kids what this means at this stage. The only dynamic I can discover is that it covers a wide gamut of possible activities, including simply being identified as a couple by others in the group. It certainly does refer to intense feelings of sexual and emotional attraction.

Think back to our general discussion of development for babies and small children. They go through a phase in which their identity is synonymous with ours. They don't know how to separate "me" from "you." Gradually, they learn to walk and talk and explore the world for themselves. They will go through periods of rebellious behaviors ("No! I don't want to do that!") and temper tantrums in the process of establishing their own identities.

It is not much different now in adolescence. At times our kids will find it difficult to separate their identities from their group. They will seek to fit in by doing everything together with the group, with a special friend, or with a romantic interest. It is what psychologists call "being enmeshed." In the later teenage years, as we will see, they will gradually learn how to be individuals again. In seeking to identify with their group or their friends, their separation from us will continue. Sometimes they will seem to have intense and loyal attachments to us. At other times they will be rebellious and defiant and act as if they don't even know us.

Although they need the physical comforts of home, adolescents will develop strong urges to be independent. Suddenly they may not want to do anything with you anymore. As your child seems to be "leaving" emotionally, you may find that your own adolescent memories of not fitting in are triggered. My family loved going to the movies. I remember the day when I simply didn't want to be seen with my parents at the show anymore but couldn't explain why. Adolescents will be testing their independence and their limits. If they didn't develop self-confidence at earlier ages, they may not know how to negotiate their need for independence. Of course, parents worry about them, so a battle ensues for control of the reins.

This stage of parenting will be confusing for you and may even be dangerous if you view this behavior as being about their love for you. It isn't. Be careful to monitor you own adolescent feelings of rejection and abandonment. Make sure you find support from your spouse, accountability group, or friends. Don't let your outlook on life be dependent on whether or not your children even seem to like you during this stage. Try not to shame or embarrass them for the things they do. They are still looking for love, touch, and affirmation from you. If you are tempted to think that your child, at this age, can be your best friend, look at your own issues about needing friendship.

Ruth's mother seemed to really enjoy being with her. Every day after school, she wanted to know what Ruth had done at school and what her friends had gossiped about. Ruth's mom liked to exchange clothes with her. She took her on long shopping expeditions to the mall and gloried in the fact that their sizes were nearly the same. It embarrassed Ruth to death that even at church her mom looked like one of her friends. Ruth's mom would pour her heart out to her daughter about her own feelings and her relationship with Ruth's dad, including their sexual relationship. Ruth's mom said that she hoped it would be helpful for Ruth to hear these things. Ruth felt sorry for her dad. Then one day Ruth came home from school to find her mom reading one of her diaries. She was mortified.

Ruth's mom is in trouble. She is lonely and trying to find a best friend in her own daughter. She has crossed many healthy and safe boundaries. She is possessing, not nurturing, her daughter. If she doesn't learn how to examine her own needs for relationship and how to get them met in healthy ways, she will continue to make it difficult for her daughter to individuate and form healthy relationships with her peers.

Dating and Sexual Experimentation

In addition to the task of beginning to separate from one's identity with parents and to find identity as an individual, children in this age group attach to friends and community to find acceptance and approval in a larger community. An adolescent may seek to form his or her identity by being valued or loved by another. Two young people may become very attached to each other, just as a child feels very attached to her parents. The couple may confuse their strong emotional and physical feelings with being in love. With hormonal attraction running rampant and their deep emotional needs to feel loved and attached, adolescents find it easy to believe that their physical feelings of attraction need to be expressed. At this point boys and girls will have to be taught how to moderate and control those feelings.

Beth and David, both age twelve, really liked each other. They were in many of the same classes at school. They went to the same church youth group. Both had begun to develop physically. At a seventh-grade dance, they danced all the slow dances together and felt those feelings of physical attraction that can be so powerful at this age. They decided to "go together."

Beth and David lived within walking distance of each other's homes. David's parents felt that he was old enough now to occasionally stay by himself, so one evening they went out on a date and left David alone in the house. That night, Beth told her parents that she was going over to her girlfriend's house but went to David's instead. They watched TV and listened to music and felt those magical feelings of unbounded attraction. As the night went on, they began to kiss. It was the first time for both of them, and it felt really wonderful. Caught up in the moment, David's natural inclination was to begin to explore this exciting thing, the female body. Beth wanted to be touched and felt really close to David, but there was something inside of her that worried about what they were doing.

When David's parents came home earlier than they had planned, they discovered Beth and David on the couch. Beth was rushing to put her blouse back on.

How many of you remember moments like this? On one hand, this is a normal situation, one in which Beth and David's feelings are very natural. On the other hand, it is a very difficult moral situation. Both of them have defied well-defined boundaries established by their parents. I imagine that Beth's friends are covering for her and would have claimed to be with her if her parents had investigated. This is one of those teachable moments when the opportunity to impart a clear message should not be lost, but the fragile egos of these two must not be damaged.

We don't know all the sexual messages that Beth and David have learned. We can assume that they have been exposed to many, both positive and negative, from a variety of sources, reliable and otherwise.

There is an old belief that the girl may be more in control of situations like the one in which Beth and David found themselves. This idea is partly due to the reality that a boy's sexual drive expresses itself faster and takes less time to get into full gear. In that sense, a girl may have a greater ability to put the brakes on. Even so, boys have to be taught to avoid getting into tempting situations. In David's case, inviting a girl to be alone with him at his house was going too far.

The situation with Beth and David prompted several conversations. David's parents talked to both children before taking Beth home and informing her parents of the facts.

"We're sorry to walk in on you like this," they said kindly. "This kind of surprise is embarrassing. We're disappointed that you both felt you had to be together without telling us about it. We know that you like each other very much, and that is a good thing. We have a rule in this house that David is not to have any friends over when we're not here. Beth, we think you're a wonderful girl, but it was wrong for you to come over here. We'll take you home and your parents can talk to you there."

When they returned, David's parents talked to him alone.

"Son, you have violated one of the house rules, and there will be a punishment for that. What you did is deceitful and we can't ignore that, but we also want you to know that we understand that many kids are doing this and it must be hard for you not to. We know that you have very strong feelings about Beth. She is a sweet girl and very attractive. It is a wonderful thing to experience those feelings. Some of those feelings are sexual and that is perfectly normal. What you did tonight is the result of putting yourself in a situation in which it is hard to resist those feelings. We don't want you to stop being with Beth, but we do need to talk about healthy ways to do that without putting yourself in inappropriate situations."

David's dad continued the conversation with him later.

"Son, I certainly remember what it is like to have your first girlfriend and to have a lot of really intense feelings for her. Tonight your sexual feelings must have been pretty strong. I also know what that is like. You are going to have those feelings a lot, so it is time for you to learn how to deal with them.

"Mom and I want it to be your choice to not fully express those feelings until you get married. We know that we can't make that decision for you. We believe that it is

God's plan for you to wait. God is not trying to spoil all the fun; he is just pointing us to really great feelings of fulfillment when we do get married. God has designed the relationship of one man and one woman in marriage to be very special, and sex is part of that one-of-a-kind specialness.

"If you're going to wait, there will be lots of times when you are frustrated. If you make that decision, a lot of times you will feel left out because it will seem that many of your friends are being sexual. I wish there was a switch that we could turn off in our brains that would prevent us from having sexual feelings until we get married, but there isn't.

"You may be frustrated tonight and even feel angry with Mom and me for coming home early. You might be angry that you didn't get to continue with Beth. You are probably wondering and worried about Beth and her parents. Mom and I hope that you can talk to her soon."

At Beth's house, the conversation went something like this.

"We know that this is a really embarrassing moment for you," her parents said. "It is not easy to be brought home by your boyfriend's parents. We also know that you really like David, and you really wanted to be with him. He is a great boy and we like him a lot too. But we are angry that you chose to deceive us. That is a violation of our rules, and there will be some consequences."

Beth's parents were surprised by all of the old "tapes" that were running through their heads from when they were adolescents. Beth's mom heard the voice of her mother telling her to be wary of boys who only wanted sex. Beth's dad heard his mother saying to him that nice girls wouldn't come over to your house. Both of them felt all of the old anxieties about sexuality that they had experienced. Beth's dad felt lots of anger about aggressive boys, remembering what he had been like. Beth's mom felt worried: Could her twelve-year-old "little girl" get pregnant? So they were both tempted to say lots of things that would have been voices from the past.

"Beth, we need to calm down a little and talk with each other about this situation and about what kind of punishment we will give you for deceiving us. But we want you to know that we understand. We remember times like this for us when we

were your age. Even though we're angry, we really love you and we do understand. We're glad that you have found a boy who really likes you. We know that your curiosity and feelings about love and about sex are running high. You already know how we feel about God's plan for sexuality, and we hope that you will decide to wait until you're married to be completely sexual. Right now, though, you are probably more worried about what everyone else is thinking and embarrassed about being discovered.

"We're sure you understand that we need to know where you are. It is as much a matter of safety as anything else. Just as we always let you know what we're doing, we hope that you will feel that same responsibility to keep us informed about you. It is our job to protect you. We ask you to respect our feelings just as we try to respect yours."

Later, Beth's mom talked to her further.

"I know that tonight was probably a wonderful night for you for a while. It is always exciting to feel like you're in love. I remember some of the boys that I felt like I was in love with. They were almost all I could think about for long periods of time. I would write their names in a school notebook a thousand times and would do anything I thought I needed to do to get their attention. You are a beautiful young woman. Boys will be attracted to your body and your wonderful smile. If it is your decision to wait until you get married to have sexual intercourse (and your father and I pray it is), you will need to avoid certain situations. When your sexual energy gets going past a certain level, it is really hard to stop."

In all of the above conversations, David's and Beth's parents are affirming their children's growing independence and sexual development while they are also enforcing the family rules and honest expressing their feelings of anger and disappointment. As parents, they recognize that any feelings from their youth are their responsibility to discuss with each other and not necessarily with their children. They take seriously their responsibility to teach their kids a biblical perspective on sexuality: "For you know what instructions we gave you by the authority of the Lord Jesus. It is God's will that you should be sanctified: that you should avoid sexual immorality; that each of you should learn to control his own body in a way that is holy and honorable, not in passionate lust like the heathen, who do not know God" (1 Thessalonians 4:2-5). These families will need to have more conversations about this situation and similar ones. Here are some general guidelines about what needs to be said:

- Sexual feelings are normal and will seek to be expressed.
- Sex does not equal love. Feeling sexual toward someone does not mean you are in love with them.
- Feeling emotionally attached is not the same as being in love.
- You will feel like you are in love and deeply committed to another person, but until you are older these feelings are difficult to trust. Emotions fluctuate so much at this age that they must be treated carefully.
- In God's design, sexual intercourse is reserved for marriage.
- Not being sexual is a positive choice to wait for something more fulfilling and special.
- When you are alone with someone of the opposite sex, it is hard to resist your emotional and sexual feelings.
- You will have to plan ahead to avoid tempting situations.
- You will feel left out if you don't participate in what everyone else seems to be doing.
- Find friends who share your values.

This last message is crucial. Kids at these ages are strongly influenced by what their friends are doing. They need to feel like they belong, so it is important to help them find communities of friends with similar morals and values. Friendship and support are the key. Feeling lonely, left out, unattractive, or unpopular are common feelings at this age, and they leave adolescents dangerously vulnerable to all sorts of peer pressure, including pressure to be sexual.

Parents need to be careful not to place so many restrictions on adolescents that their feelings of loneliness increase. We must proactively look for ways to help our children feel loved and included. Touching them in healthy ways, affirming them for whatever success or accomplishment, and complimenting them on their appearance are vital preventive strategies for this stage.

HEALTHY SEXUALITY DURING PUBERTY: PERSONAL DIMENSION

The personal dimension of healthy sexuality is more specific than just the personal identity described earlier. It is about one's sense of self as a person and as a sexual being. The dimensions overlap during this stage. The many physical, emotional, and spiritual developments of this stage affect a child's personal identity. Our young adolescents' abilities to know and like themselves physically, to express their feelings honestly, to relate to others in healthy ways, and to have a relationship with God are all critical to having a healthy sense of self. The crucial work in the personal dimension at this stage will be built on healthy development in all the dimensions at earlier ages.

Two major developmental issues in the personal dimension are key during this stage. The first is whether a healthy sense of one's sexual self exists and is developing normally. The second involves one's sense of sexual orientation.

Healthy Sexual Identity Versus Sexual Shame

Like most people who have psychological training, I tend to think in terms of problems that can develop. Let's start with a brief look at those and then try to characterize a young adolescent who has a healthy sexual identity.

Sexual shame develops when children think they are bad people, that no one will love them, and that no one finds them attractive. In my first book, *Faithful and True: Sexual Integrity in a Fallen World,* I describe two forms of trauma that can create this sense of sexual shame in adolescents. First, a child can be emotionally, physically, or sexually invaded. This means that horrible things have happened to the child. We characterize these things by using the word *abuse.* I believe that such invasion has an emotional and spiritual effect. Second, a child can be abandoned—that is, his or her basic needs for emotional, physical, sexual, and spiritual nurture are not met. These kids have not been affirmed, touched, given healthy sexual information, or taught and modeled sound spiritual truth. This form of trauma can also be profoundly abusive.

In chapter 5 I briefly described the symptoms of sexual abuse or invasion. By the time your child reaches puberty, you might have seen some of these. In later adolescence, others may appear, such as getting involved in some form of addictive sexual activity, being totally turned off to sex, or getting involved in unhealthy relationships. If you are noticing any of these signs, you may need to consult with a skilled counselor who can help diagnose the problem and offer you options for helping your child find healing.

The important point is that a person who has suffered invasion trauma, and therefore feels sexual shame, will seek to find relief for that shame. Sometimes this will involve acting in sexual ways that repeat the early trauma with the hope that the hurt will go away. For example, a child may get involved in relationships with people who are like the person who originally invaded him or her. Or the child may act in sexually aggressive ways, thinking that this means having control over sex. A child who has been abandoned may turn to sex, thinking that it is the only way he or she will be loved and touched. Many voices in our culture teach this message. Finally, the child may totally turn off sexual feelings, again as an attempt to be in control of sex.

This is only a brief introduction to this complex topic. I would not include it in a book for all parents if I did not know how common these problems are. I hope and pray that you can almost skip over this section and the next because your kids don't have these problems. If you are, however, seeing some basic symptoms of dysfunctional sexual behaviors, get some help; don't try to diagnose these yourself. This chapter and others offer enough stories of sexual abuse that you should get a good idea of what to look for.

If you have been having effective conversations with your kids about sex throughout their childhood, their chances of developing a healthy sense of themselves will be much higher. Below is a list of characteristics you will begin to see in your children at this age if they are developing healthy sexuality:

- will feel physically attractive
- are comfortable in social relationships with both males and females
- will not be frightened by the thought of sex
- may experiment with some forms of sexual thought and activity but will not get stuck in repetitive patterns with any of them. From any experimentation that they may do, they will learn, mature, and come to make healthy moral choices.
- are involved in relationships that are mutual, not dependent or abusive in any way

Homosexuality

Roy and Jerry were very good friends who grew up together. They both liked music, computers, and playing chess. They didn't like sports very much. In many ways they didn't exemplify ruggedly male characteristics. They loved being with each other and talked and talked. They didn't think about girls much. Some of their friends saw the intensity of their relationship and started calling them "fags." Their minister at church was always preaching against homosexuality and found ways of including it in almost every sermon. This made both of them feel really different and alone. They came to depend on their friendship even more.

One night around age thirteen, while sleeping over at one of their houses, they experimented with masturbating each other. It felt good to them, and they continued it. They began to conclude that they must be gay.

These two boys genuinely love each other as friends. They experience *philia* love for each other, so it is not unnatural for them to want to touch each other. But they crossed a boundary when they became sexual with each other. It felt good physically, so they have reached the logical conclusion that they are homosexual. Notice, however, that what drives them deeper into their homosexual feelings is the relationship in which they find true acceptance and the experience of physical nurturing. That observation could give any of us some clues about what kids really need. The path to being a healthy heterosexual might include that much-needed sense of acceptance and physical touch.

Feeling confused about sexual attraction is not abnormal as adolescents explore their sexual feelings and their friendships with members of the same sex as well as of the opposite sex. If a child is labeled a homosexual by his peers early in life, the rejection and isolation may drive him deeper into the experience. Many homosexual people believe that they were born that way. They are sincerely convinced that they have no choice because their feelings of being different and of being attracted to the same sex go back as far as they can remember. I have talked to countless people struggling with very real anguish because they have tried unsuccessfully to be heterosexual; they have prayed and truly sought not to be gay. Many of them have felt condemned and ostracized by the church. Many Christians don't understand the sincerity of their efforts to change and believe that they simply have made an immoral choice.

Before I discuss the issue of homosexuality any further, please know that I recognize how controversial this topic is. Many Christians and non-Christians alike interpret Scripture and doctrine differently on this issue. On both sides of the debate, rigid black-and-white thinking has resulted in people not talking to each other. It seems to me that this is the worst result.

Please accept my own thoughts on this issue as the fruit of prayerful struggle. I don't have all the answers, but the teaching of the Bible seems quite clear on homosexuality. In 1 Corinthians 6:9 the apostle Paul includes homosexuality on his list of sexually immoral behaviors. Many other scriptures in both the Old and New Testament speak of homosexual behavior as a sexual sin and as an abomination to God. My feeling is that God is not saying no to homosexual behavior just because it's different from the norm. My understanding of Scripture leads me to believe that God's plan for sexuality is represented in the sacred one-flesh nature of the marriage of a man and a woman. This is God's order for the world. As Paul taught, a mystical union occurs between a man and a woman when they consummate their committed love relationship. It is a completion, a fulfillment.

Another reason I believe that homosexual behavior can be labeled as sinful is that it seems to fall short of God's highest vision for our personal fulfillment. The following definition of sin applies across the board: Any behavior that alienates us from God and from each other is sin. So is anything that creates chaos in the moral order and in God's plan for the universe. These are the standards by which I believe we must judge whether or not homosexual behavior is sinful.

Scientifically, the issue of the genetic origin of homosexuality has never been proven. For years researchers have tried to isolate a gene or a genetic marker that causes homosexuality. Studies that have supposedly demonstrated a genetic link have failed to be duplicated in similar studies. At this point, there simply is no conclusive evidence that homosexuality is an unavoidable choice. Even some of the most vocal supporters of homosexuality admit that how a child is raised must be taken into account in the development of homosexuality. Some researchers believe that any genetic predisposition to same-sex orientation must be developed by complex environmental factors to result in a person being gay.

As Christians, we know that we are born with the potential for good and for evil. How we are nurtured will help to determine what choices we make later in life. However, we must be careful in our approach to the concept of choice related to sexual orientation. Since so many gay people believe they have no choice, where does the problem first occur? My belief is that the environmental factors that create homosexual behaviors can occur so early in a child's life that he or she doesn't even remember them. Also, a child is not likely to be fully conscious of the complex emotional issues involved. It does, therefore, seem to them that they never made any decision. Long and complicated therapy may be needed to help them sort out the truth.

This topic of whether or not homosexual orientation can be "repaired" is, however, very controversial. Homosexuality is no longer labeled as a medical or psychiatric disease. The American Psychiatric Association recently said that to even counsel a person to change is unethical. Therapists are being sued for trying to do so. Some Christians, on the other hand, think that simply repenting is enough to change a person's orientation.

Research has shown that the human brain creates its own message pathways linking how a person thinks and feels to how he reacts biologically. It is possible that when a developing person consistently repeats homosexual behaviors, the brain adjusts itself to the fact that this is the pattern, believes it to be true, and calls for more and more similar thoughts to achieve the same sexual feeling.

Emotional factors that might contribute to a homosexual orientation are more complex. A commonly held view among Christian therapists is that, developmentally, children and adolescents who are homosexually oriented haven't learned how to form healthy attachments with the same-sex parent. Another theory is that some children who have been sexually abused suffer a blow to their sexual development that can contribute to a homosexual orientation.

With all the controversy, hostility, and fear that currently infuses the social and political debate on these issues, it's tempting for parents to either avoid discussing the subject of homosexuality with their children or to overreact to what are actually normal parts of a child's developmental process. For example, children who engage in same-sex sexual play with kids of the same age are probably just experimenting with their own bodies and not with homosexuality. Like the boys in our stories, kids may be experimenting within very special friendships with members of the same sex, friendships that are intimate emotionally and sometimes physically.

As we talk with our children about what we believe is healthy sexuality, we must be open to listening to their internal struggles as they encounter the various thoughts and feelings related to sexuality during this tumultuous stage. While we are stating our own beliefs, we must seek to love and accept our children no matter what they may be experiencing. Anger and rejection may only push them deeper into their pain and loneliness.

Robert, age thirteen, was genuinely frightened. He felt himself to be different somehow. He liked girls but mainly for their sensitive personalities. He didn't like the competitiveness of the boys around them. He didn't find their sexual teasing and jokes all that funny. Most of all, he didn't find the thought of females to be that sexually stimulating. He embarrassed himself a number of times by having an erection in the locker room when he saw some of the boys naked. Robert excelled in drama and music. Some of the kids teased him about being a "fag."

Robert's dad encouraged him to be more like a "man." His dad worked a lot and drank. When he was drunk, he was often full of rage. Robert's mom cowered in her husband's presence. She took out her anger and frustration on Robert and sought to control every aspect of his life. He didn't know who to talk to about his feelings. Finally, one day he confessed his thoughts to one of his teachers who had always seemed more sensitive than the rest. This teacher referred Robert to a group of teens who were meeting to discuss the issue of homosexuality and offer each other support. When Robert entered that room and heard the discussion, he finally felt like he was "home."

Robert is in trouble at the same time he is finally finding support and acceptance. Attending the gay students' support group is not helping him deal with the painful issues with his parents, which are even older than his feelings of being gay. He has never felt accepted for who he is. His dad never gave him affirmation and his mom sought to control his life. His God-given gifts are not what culture values as being "manly." Who will accept him for who he is, not overreact to his homosexual feelings, and seek to guide him to the kind of help he needs? If he ever "comes out" to his parents and they get angry, Robert will feel more rejection, and this will push him even farther away from exploring the roots of his homosexual feelings.

Eric was a lot like Robert. His dad died when he was three, and his mom did the best she could to raise him. She later married a man who tried but wasn't very good at being a father. Eric had lots of talents and abilities that weren't well accepted by his friends. He acted in certain "feminine" ways. He was sensitive and gifted but also easily hurt and wounded. He was aware of being attracted to boys very early in his life. Eric's mom took him to a skilled Christian counselor and pastor when he was ten. Here are some of the things this pastor said to him:

"Eric, you are a wonderful young man. You have many God-given talents. Many people will come to love you for being so sensitive and caring. I know that it has been really tough for you. You have had a hard life. Your dad died. Your mom has had to work a lot and hasn't been around. Your stepdad is a good man, but no one can replace your biological father.

"I want you to know that you may be having feelings of attraction to boys or to men. You are very vulnerable to needing the healthy physical touch of a man. You need a man to be caring, accepting, affirming, and available to you. I want you to know that you can find these things, but they don't have to be sexually expressed."

This is only a beginning conversation. More than that, it is the beginning of an ongoing conversation that may lead this counselor to be a healthy "father figure" in Eric's life. He will still have to work on his feelings of sexual attraction to the same sex. He may need specialized counseling. But the first step to helping Eric is to surround him with safety and grace.

My suggestion is that you have the kind of conversations with your child that could be briefly summarized by this one:

"We have already talked about the fact that, as you become a man (or a woman), you will develop feelings of sexual attraction. These are both exciting and scary. All people are different as to how intense these feelings will be. Sometimes they will be so intense it will seem like you are on fire. One of the scariest things that can happen is that you may have feelings of sexual attraction to the same sex. This can be very normal. The main thing we want you to know is that we accept and love you for whatever feelings you have. We commit to you that we will not be angry with you for coming

to talk to us about whatever is going on inside you. We also commit to not judging you or condemning you in any way. But this does not mean that we accept certain behaviors. We believe that expressing sexual feelings outside a marriage relationship can lead to very destructive patterns. Finally, we commit to helping you deal with any feelings you have. We will get you help and support you as you continue to develop into the man (or woman) God has designed you to be."

Like all the conversations in this book, this example is meant to serve as a model for longer and ongoing conversations. If your child has come to you with feelings of homosexual attraction, find a skilled counselor who can lovingly get to the root of any emotional problems that might be going on. You could be threatened by this, thinking that it may be a poor reflection on your parenting skills. It might, but be of good courage. Having a child come to you about these things doesn't necessarily mean that you are a bad parent or that he or she has been sexually abused. But by getting help now, you will prevent major problems in the future. In the next chapter, I will address the issue of what to say if your teenager comes to you and says that he or she is gay.

HEALTHY SEXUALITY DURING PUBERTY: SPIRITUAL DIMENSION

During this stage of development, boys and girls often will act like children and then at other times surprise us by how mature they are. As Paul taught in 1 Corinthians 13, one of the challenges of this transitional stage is to stop thinking like a child and to develop spiritual maturity. On the other hand, as Jesus taught, unless we become like little children, at least spiritually, we can never inherit the kingdom of God.

With children becoming rather defiant about being independent and having control of their own lives, it will be challenging and frustrating at times to guide them toward the kind of spiritual maturity that both Paul and Jesus talked about. Cultural influences will tempt children to act like adults prematurely. Of course, their peers will influence them to conform and be like everyone else. Some of this pressure will be exhibited in sexual ways.

Spiritually, young adolescents will seek to fit in with their peer group. They probably will be more attracted to the church youth group if popular kids belong to it. But even if they have accepted Christ as their Savior, they will still be rather vulnerable to what others think. On one hand, in their search for independence, adolescents may rebel against the rigid black-and-white answers they have grown up with. On the other hand, they may be attracted to those religious disciplines that give them rigid black-and-white answers different from what they have known. This is a time when adolescents are dangerously vulnerable to cults and other false religions. It is also a time, however, when their intense desire to belong and to be part of something important to them can help draw them closer to God.

One of the tasks for parents at this stage is to direct children to spiritual authorities who are trustworthy. In 3 John 11, John reminded his readers that imitating others who are godly is a healthy discipline. One of the best ways to teach this to your children is to model trustworthy behavior. Do what you say you're going to do. Be consistent in your behaviors. Practice spiritual disciplines as individuals, as a couple, and as a family. When you are wrong, admit it and try to make things right. Be accountable and tell your kids how you're doing so.

Your children will also need to be around other healthy role models. In order for this to happen, you may have to surrender being the main spiritual influence in your child's life. Either now in early adolescence or in later teenage years, you need to accept that many others can have a wonderful spiritual influence on your child.

Think about the people who have been the most powerful spiritual influences in your life. Who were your mentors? One of the best ways to help your children find spiritual mentors of their own is to send them to safe spiritual environments like church, concerts, youth rallies, or church camps. Allow them to find trustworthy guides for themselves.

Lisa's parents showed her a list of church camps that their denomination was sponsoring in various parts of the country. They said, "We think that it would be great for you to go to one of these. We will pay for it. We would like you to choose which place sounds like the most fun to you. Maybe you would like to check with some of your friends to see if they would want to go with you."

These parents are making it possible for their daughter to gain positive spiritual direction in a fun environment with her peers. They basically trust their denomination to provide good leadership. They have talked to other parents who have sent their kids to these camps before and have heard that it was a good experience. They are giving their daughter the choice of exactly where to go and possibly who to go with. At one of these camps, Lisa will find Christian mentors who model healthy spiritual development.

HEALTHY SEXUALITY CHECKLIST

Before your child enters late adolescence, he or she should have accomplished several developmental tasks during puberty.

Physical. Children should understand the basic biology of sex and reproduction, how their bodies are changing, and that variations in how quickly or slowly these changes take place are common. Parents should be sensitive to children's physical insecurities during this stage and offer plenty of affirmation.

Emotional. Children should be aware of what different feelings are like and have some experience in expressing them. They should know that there are unhealthy substitutes for intimacy and be aware of what some of those are. Parents should assure children that puberty is an emotionally volatile time and that this is normal.

Relational. Children should begin to experience sexual feelings of attraction and know that these are normal. They should understand the nature of friendship and begin to experience it with both males and females one on one as well as in groups. Parents should monitor their children's experimentation with the opposite sex, teaching healthy boundaries without overreacting to normal behaviors.

Personal. Children should recognize their own worth, like themselves as people, and be free from the pain of past wounds. Parents should help them deal with any feelings of shame or confusion about sexuality and sexual orientation.

Spiritual. Children should be exposed in the family and outside of it to positive spiritual authorities, disciplines, and influences. They need to have some freedom to ask their own questions. Fitting in socially in religious settings will be important, and parents should help facilitate positive religious experiences in community.

As you will see in the next chapter, if some of these developmental tasks are not accomplished during this stage (which is not uncommon), they will manifest themselves in later teenage years. By its very nature adolescence is a turbulent time—a crucial time in which unhealthy or healthy patterns will be established, sometimes for the rest of a person's life. Take a deep breath. Talk to other parents. Pray a lot. Be gentle with yourself.

I am aware that sometimes when I talk or write about these things, parents come down really hard on themselves for mistakes they think they have already made with their children. You probably have made some mistakes, as we all do. But remember that most kids are resilient and very forgiving. They need you to love them, and they need you to correct any mistakes that you are currently making. They may even need you to apologize, particularly as they get older. You are doing the best that you know how to do. If you have problems changing some of your negative behaviors, get some help for yourself.

Now tighten your emotional seat belt because we're moving on to the rest of the teenage years.

CHAPTER SEVEN

Adolescence

(A G E   1 5 – 1 9)

Lynn and Don, age seventeen, had been going together for several months. They really liked each other and had come to depend on their relationship to meet most of their social needs. They both came from Christian families and had been raised in the church. Neither had experienced any major developmental problems, and both seemed to be doing well in school and in other aspects of their lives.

Lynn and Don knew that many of their friends were experimenting with various sexual behaviors. Up to now they themselves had not ventured past lots of kissing and cuddling. They went to movies together, listened to music on the radio, hung out at each other's houses, and watched TV. They were great companions. They discussed their plans for college and their dreams for the future. In some ways, they were feeling very grown-up and ready to enter life after high school.

One night in the car after seeing a movie, their making out became very passionate. Some touching happened that hadn't happened before. Lynn drew back after a while and sighed, "I don't know that we should be doing this." Various messages from her parents and her church were going through her head. She was also frightened. Don was frustrated and overwhelmed by the feelings he was having at the moment. "Lynn, there's nothing to be afraid of. We're old enough to make this decision. God knows we care about each other." Lynn felt deeply about Don, and she didn't want him to be mad at her. She didn't know what to do.

YOUR CHILD'S BASIC DEVELOPMENTAL TASKS

Most teenagers experiment quite a bit during this stage as they explore the differences between friendship and romance. Culturally, they are being bombarded with sexual stimuli and temptation. They may feel rather left out if they are not sexually experienced.

The teenage years are usually a less volatile time than puberty and early adolescence in terms of the five aspects of development described in the healthy sexuality model in chapter 2. Many of the issues teens confront, however, are the same as those of the previous stage, except at a more advanced level.

Our children's primary job during the teenage years is to continue to form their own identities. As they mature, their personal identities will be less defined by outside approval or by being part of a particular group. The friction and tension that often arise between parents and children during this stage are a result of the teenagers' need to exercise their growing independence. They will usually seek to detach from their dependence on mom and dad, and they may choose to experiment more with various behavioral choices.

Your child's primary developmental tasks during later adolescence include the following:

- accepting the uniqueness of his or her own body, its attractiveness, and what it needs to be healthy
- understanding the specifics of all aspects of sexuality, including problems that can develop
- knowing how to deal with complex and difficult feelings and being able to express them appropriately
- understanding that some ways of dealing with moods and feelings are inappropriate
- developing friendships with males and females in which they can share their feelings deeply

- knowing what a safe relationship is like with members of the opposite sex
- building healthy communities of friends in various church and social situations
- having a positive sense of who they are, including their sexuality
- developing their own relationship with God
- embracing a vision of God's plan for their lives, including the possibility of marriage and family
- drawing on God's power to achieve spiritual goals
- understanding God's grace, particularly in light of any mistakes they have made

YOUR PRIMARY PARENTING TASKS

As children sprout the wings of adolescence, some parents find it difficult to let go and not be too controlling. Not only do we worry about them, but we also are adjusting to a significant change in our own lives. For many of us, our lives have revolved around our children for so long that we may experience a profound sense of sadness or loneliness. When parents are having a hard time letting their teens individuate in a healthy way, friction increases. So one of our jobs as parents is to let our teenagers become more independent while continuing to enforce healthy spiritual, physical, and emotional boundaries in the home.

Conversations during this stage should involve talking to our kids further about sexual abstinence before marriage and the spiritual and emotional value of doing so. We can't just scare them about sexually transmitted diseases or possible unwanted pregnancies. We must be willing to offer them solid biblical reasons why it is important to wait, how they will honor their future spouses if they do, and why the sexual relationship in marriage is not only sacred but also positive and fulfilling.

We should also engage our teenagers in practical conversations about dealing with peer pressure or a boyfriend or girlfriend who is sexually aggressive. It is a time to let our kids know more about our struggles with these various temptations and to remind them that we will always be a resource for them.

For some parents the greatest challenge of this stage may be just to *have* a conversation. Often, parents will need to pray for other adults or authority figures to be positive role models for their kids.

To summarize, your primary tasks as you parent your teenager include the following:

- Continue conversation at all levels while at the same time allowing your child to be more in control of it.
- Teach about specific sexual behaviors and problems.
- Model healthy thought, behavior, and communication.
- Affirm your children in all aspects of their lives.
- Set safe boundaries for your children.
- Encourage them to be spiritually and socially active.
- Be aware of any behavioral problems or unhealthy patterns and find help if needed.
- Challenge them with spiritual vision.
- Model God's grace.

Before we look in more detail at the specific developmental issues our teenagers face, let's remember that as parents we will all make mistakes with our kids. I have known parents who are paralyzed by the fear that they might do the wrong thing. One antidote to fear is to realize that we "*all* have sinned and fall short of the glory of God" (Romans 3:23, emphasis added). Nobody is perfect, and God doesn't expect us to be perfect parents. God does want us to persevere, however, through all the ups and downs:

> Not only so, but we also rejoice in our sufferings, because we know that suffering produces perseverance; perseverance, charac-

ter; and character, hope. And hope does not disappoint us, because God has poured out his love into our hearts by the Holy Spirit, whom he has given us.

You see, at just the right time, when we were still powerless, Christ died for the ungodly. (Romans 5:3-6)

If we persevere, even when parenting produces suffering, we will develop character, which produces hope. Hope never disappoints us. You may often feel powerless because your kids don't always make the right decisions, at least as far as you're concerned. But that powerlessness can be a reminder that God is in control and that Jesus died even for the ungodly decisions of those you love the most.

Years ago my dad told me something that I still carry with me. He said a day never goes by when he doesn't pray for me. While he made some mistakes as a parent that have affected me, he gave me a wonderful gift when, each day, he turned me over to my heavenly Father. Always remember that, when your teenagers are often out there by themselves in our pressure-filled world, praying for them is one of the best things you can do for them—and for yourself—as you continue to surrender control of their lives to a loving God.

HEALTHY SEXUALITY DURING ADOLESCENCE: PHYSICAL DIMENSION

During adolescence, the body is completing the process of becoming an adult. Some children will be fully developed by this stage, while others won't. My son Jon was always rather small for his age. Then in his junior year of high school he grew six inches in three months and was one of the tallest kids in his class. Think of the wardrobe adjustments alone! But many other adjustments to one's developing body can also be challenging during this stage.

Attractiveness

While this is the time when young people are at the height of their sexual attraction to each other, be aware that the battle about feeling personally attractive has not necessarily been resolved. The memories of the embarrassment of acne or of being too short, fat, tall, or thin may still be painful for your kids. The teasing from earlier years may still be sounding in their ears. Additionally, cultural influences may be influencing teenagers about what they should look like. If you haven't done so lately, pick up some of the magazines geared toward teenagers and notice the messages they communicate about physical appearance.

Adolescents sometimes struggle with powerful feelings of shame related to their physical development. I have worked with a number of young female models who have appeared on the covers of various magazines. Even though the world considers them beautiful, they have a hard time believing it.

In her younger years, Jennifer had a weight problem. It was minor; certainly no one would have called her fat, but she felt that way. Through the years she matured into a beautiful seventeen-year-old. She developed a nice figure, and in no way was she overweight. Many boys found her extremely attractive. However, Jennifer couldn't stand looking in the mirror. She thought her hips were too wide, her breasts too large. So she went on a diet. Even after reaching her initial weight-loss goal, she still didn't like the way she looked.

Teenagers can set the stage for a variety of physical problems by trying to appear physically attractive to each other. Eating disorders are common, especially among girls. Boys, too, can get into this kind of trouble. The use of drugs to enhance bodybuilding is another dangerous temptation. If teenagers are ashamed of their physical appearance, trying to look sexier and acting out sexually can also appear to be an antidote. The main point is, even if you think your teenager is attractive—and others do too—he or she may not think so. Your teenager may need some specific help in talking through his or her own self-perceptions. One goal in this stage is to help your child value his or her body as much more than a means of attracting the opposite sex. You will need to lead conversations about the fact that physical attraction is much more than the size or shape of any body part.

Throughout adolescence, teenagers will need to be told that everyone is different and that everyone is attractive in their own way. It is not a bad time to remind them of this Bible passage:

> For you created my inmost being; you knit me together in my mother's womb. I praise you because I am fearfully and wonderfully made; your works are wonderful, I know that full well. My frame was not hidden from you when I was made in the secret place. When I was woven together in the depths of the earth, your eyes saw my unformed body. All the days ordained for me were written in your book before one of them came to be. (Psalm 139:13-16)

God made each of us different, but we are all fearfully and wonderfully made. I love that image. God knew our exact form before each of us even had a body. If God is in charge of even the smallest details of our physical being, then he is surely in control of the people out there who will be attracted to it. Reassuring your children of such truths can help to ease their anxiety about their physical appearance.

Self-care

Since God made us and our bodies are temples of the Holy Spirit (1 Corinthians 3:16), we should take care of ourselves. We should never worship our bodies, but we should treat them with honor and respect. Teenagers need to be taught how to care for their bodies. This includes getting enough sleep, eating right, exercising, and grooming. But remember, as teens practice being more independent and making decisions, they may choose to stay up all night and sleep until noon. They will eat candy bars, popcorn, and pizza. Their only concept of exercise may be sitting in the bathtub, pulling the plug, and fighting against the current.

If your teenager is less than inspirational in terms of self-care and personal motivation, accept your exasperation. It is normal parental stuff. Remember that teenagers don't respond to shame like, "You're going to be a bum." It's far better to challenge them with their dreams.

Ben was a promising basketball player. All his coaches said so. Soon after he turned fifteen, girls discovered him in a big way. Many of his classmates looked up to him, and he suddenly found himself popular. Like many adolescents, he had been slightly overweight and had lots of anxiety about being teased because of it. So he didn't really believe his popularity and was afraid of losing it. Ben decided that he didn't want to play basketball anymore and announced that he planned to stop going to practice. His mom and dad sat him down and said, "We feel that, as you become a young man, you have the right to begin to make your own choices. Playing basketball is one of those choices, but you seem to have been given a real gift in that area.

"We need you to know that we will always love you whether or not you play basketball. That is not the real issue. Many others also will love and accept you whether or not you're a great basketball player. Right now you're finding out about others liking you, especially girls. That is really important. We celebrate that with you. But we wonder if you have given up your dream of playing basketball in college. It is a hard choice when you think that you might have to disappoint those who like you by not going to all of their parties so you can practice. It takes a lot of work to be good at something even when you're really talented. If you're afraid of the friends you'll lose or worried about the time it will take, we would like to offer you the perspective that hard work always pays off. The social things that seem so important now will hardly be remembered in a few years. We will help you be disciplined if you choose to follow your dream. God honors hard work and using your physical talents to the best of your ability. We'd like you to enjoy basketball as a way of enjoying your physical gifts."

Ben may be able to verbalize his fears or even his anger about all of the demands on his time that the discipline of hard work will take. If his parents are good listeners, they may also hear from him about his old fears of being unattractive. It is really hard for a parent to convince a child that they are attractive. They need to hear it from others.

Although it may surprise you, the above conversation is really about sex, too. Ben is wondering about being attractive to girls. Examine your own myths that kids like Ben should value playing basketball as a way of being more popular with girls. Ben's parents will need to teach him about what girls are really like and what they find attractive in the opposite sex. For example, most girls really like boys who work hard and have discipline. This is not an inappropriate motivating factor for Ben.

Specific Sexual Questions

Adolescents developing into adults will have some physical growing pains and medical concerns. Their questions about bodies and sexuality may become more sophisticated and complicated. By the time they reach age fifteen, the world has bombarded them with messages about sex and relationships. Parents will need to counter these messages through an ongoing dialogue about the truth.

By now you have already explained the mechanics and biology of sex. Since your child's early years you have used a variety of biologically accurate books to do so. Now you are having ongoing conversations as specific questions or teachable moments arise. Once your child is a teenager, it is time to make sure that certain bases have been covered. At some point, your teenager may stop asking questions or may seem to not want to talk to you, but don't assume that they know everything. Let's examine the basic issues you'll want to address with your kids during this stage.

Intercourse. You probably don't know what kind of images about intercourse your teenagers may have picked up in various places. If they have seen pornography of any kind, their minds will have been filled with images of a wide variety of sexual activity. You may simply remind them that married couples may enjoy sexual intercourse in different positions and that they will take their own journey of discovery once they are married. When it comes to the specifics of sex, it is not wise to talk about your own sex life or experience. This is something very personal, and your teenager may be totally embarrassed if you get specific about yourself. Talk in generalities.

Frequency. The main reason to cover this topic now is because of the numerous cultural messages implying that couples enjoy sex every day or even several times a day. Teenagers will be filing this impression away in their minds and building expectations for the time when they do get married. This following conversation tells a teenager the truth:

A typical eighteen-year-old, Gary had watched a fair amount of TV and recently had admitted to seeing some R-rated movies. His mom and dad sat him down and went over a variety of myths that they perceived might be in those shows. They said, "You know, one of the most common misperceptions that you might be picking up is that couples have sex all the time. This is not necessarily true. All couples are different. Some have sex every day, but that is really rare. Some have sex once or twice a week. Others have sex at regular intervals much further apart than that. Many couples go through times when the frequency of sex varies. The important thing to understand about all this is that the emotional and spiritual relationship you'll have with your future spouse will be the foundation for your sexual relationship. How often you have sex will be determined by a number of factors, including honoring whatever is going on with each of you emotionally."

Orgasm. How do you explain something that is truly unlike anything else? Many of the old textbooks on sexuality said that orgasm was like sneezing. Please! But there are some similarities. A sneeze is something that the whole body gets ready for, and when it happens there is a sense of release and relaxation. But the comparison is totally inadequate because orgasm is much more. Someone said to me that it is like riding a roller coaster with all the anticipation of climbing and then the excitement when you drop or even go upside down. I'm not sure that this is an adequate comparison either, but it does get at some of the features.

As we've discussed in previous chapters, many children will have experienced orgasm through self-stimulation by the time they are teenagers. However, they may have questions about how orgasm during intercourse is different. This is an opportunity to explain that when couples work hard at emotional and spiritual intimacy, coming together as one flesh and experiencing orgasm creates a sense of being totally "connected." It can be a spiritual experience.

Parents may also need to explain that orgasm does not always occur for women and that they may have more difficulty with it during intercourse. This may be due to a variety of factors, including poor communication between the spouses about what the woman needs in order to experience orgasm. Failure to achieve orgasm is not always a result of a woman's sexual dysfunction, although it can be. Also, pornography may suggest to women that orgasm is always wild and intense. Popular culture is teaching women that they are in control of their orgasms and that they should pursue them vigorously. If parents and children are able to discuss an issue as specific as orgasm, I think it's important to mention that not all sex results in shrieking orgasm every time.

Both young men and women need to be taught that satisfying sex can happen even if orgasm doesn't always happen, that you are not more powerful if you always have one, and that you are not incompetent if you don't. Sexual intercourse is about connecting emotionally and spiritually, not just physically. In other words, sex can be fulfilling without orgasm, and we don't need to be preoccupied about the "success" of orgasm.

Sexual dysfunction. On a topic related to orgasm, it is not a bad idea to let adolescents know that sexual functioning between husband and wife is not always perfect. It is not necessary to discuss specific sexual dysfunction at length, but this is an opportunity to prepare them for the fact that healthy and fulfilling sexuality is a matter of mutual give-and-take between husband and wife and that it often takes time for them to find their own fulfilling patterns. During the course of married life, sexual and medical issues such as impotence, infertility, childbirth, menopause, or fluctuating libido may affect a couple's sex life.

Birth control. Some parents try to scare teenagers out of being sexual by warning them about the dangers of pregnancy. They also refuse to give them information about birth control as a way of reinforcing their point.

Amy's mom got pregnant at age seventeen and gave the baby up for adoption. She told her husband, Amy's dad, about it before they got married. He had been loving and supportive. Now that Amy has started dating, her mom finds it difficult not to be frightened and overprotective. She continually warns Amy about the dangers of getting pregnant, but she has never discussed with her daughter the practical means of keeping herself safe if she does become sexual. Right now, Amy doesn't even have a serious boyfriend, and she's getting really tired of her mom's obsessive warnings.

Amy's mom is a loving person who has her daughter's best interest at heart. She doesn't want Amy to make the same mistakes and suffer the same pain and regret that she has. Her obsessive warnings, however, are more about her inability to forgive herself and to grieve the baby she gave up. A part of her spirit is still stuck in her teenage years.

Many issues may prevent us from being mature parents who use more than scare tactics and obsessive control to keep our kids safe. Scare tactics about sex rarely work. Remember, you are trying to model and teach *positive* values. Simply forbidding sexual activity or continually reminding teens how dangerous it can be may only cause them to view sexual activity as a way to be rebellious or to prove their independence.

I believe that it is wise to inform teenagers about birth-control options. Hopefully, this discussion sets the stage for making healthy decisions about when to have children after marriage. If you are facing the reality that your teenager is already sexually active, you will want to let him or her know about the pill, condoms, and other forms of birth control. You can strongly disagree with their decision about being sexually active, but by this stage in their lives you have to realize you cannot force them to obey your teaching. Being overly controlling during this time could push your child in the opposite direction you intended. Many Christian parents will disagree about giving their kids access to birth control. Some feel that it is better to provide them plenty of information about safe sex, while others feel that to do so would encourage them to be immoral. Nothing in the studies I have seen or in my experience would suggest that the latter is true. If you are confident in your teaching and in the ideals you have promoted, err on the side of helping your kids to stay safe.

Sexually transmitted diseases (STDs). As with birth control, scare tactics will not be effective in keeping your teenager safe from sexually transmitted diseases. While every parent's worst terror is that a child will contract the deadly AIDS virus, simply forbidding sexual activity may not keep the child safe. I believe that making sure teenagers have a clear understanding of various types of STDs and how they are contracted is often the best preventive measure parents can take. Here's how Rita's parents handled a discussion about STDs.

"Rita, you know that we don't think that scaring you is the right approach to convincing you to wait until you're married to be sexual, but given all the attention that the AIDS virus gets, along with other sexually transmitted diseases, we thought it would be a good idea to talk. With all the publicity, you may already know a lot about STDs. You probably know that these diseases, including AIDS, can't be contracted by simply kissing, holding hands, or hugging. It has even been shown that you can share towels or laundry with people who have AIDS and you won't get infected.

"Most STDs are spread through genital contact with a person who is already infected. This means that sexual contact with anyone who has had previous sexual experience is risky. The result may be simply that you need to get a shot of antibiotics. Or it could mean that you will contract a disease that you will carry for life. Some STDs can be controlled but not cured. You would have to use protection for the rest of your life so as not to give it to your spouse. Obviously, you would have to tell a future

spouse about any STD you have. Some STDs will create permanent damage to your genitals or reproductive organs so that you won't be able to have children. And some STDs can kill you.

"People who acquire an STD usually think it could never happen to them. We all tend to think that bad things happen to others and not to us. But we want you to be very aware that it can happen to anyone who is sexually active, so we hope that you'll continue to make godly decisions for your life. If you ever find yourself in trouble, please remember that we are here for you, and we want to make sure you get whatever help you need."

This conversation is not that lengthy or scientifically detailed. As with most conversations you'll have with your kids about sex-related issues, it emphasizes the basics and keeps things as simple as possible. If your teenager asks lots of questions and you find that you need to give a lot more specific information about STDs, you can get some help from your doctor. Obviously, if your teenager seems really curious or anxious about these things, you will want to gently investigate why this is so.

HEALTHY SEXUALITY DURING ADOLESCENCE: EMOTIONAL DIMENSION

Erik Erikson, one of the more famous developmental psychologists of this century, said that adolescence is the time when a person learns how to be either intimate or isolated. As I explained in chapter 2, intimacy is an ability to be vulnerable, to let someone else really know you. Developing this ability becomes complicated if a person has unresolved childhood and adolescent issues related to feeling unlovable. One of the major blocks to intimacy is the feeling that "If you knew me, you wouldn't like me. I'm not a lovable person." Parents will need to continue monitoring their child's "self-talk" during adolescence and encourage the sharing of feelings so self-esteem issues can be resolved.

Sharing Feelings

Being alone is not the only way human beings experience isolation. A person can be in the middle of a crowded room and be isolated because he or she is not taking the risk of being known or is not being honest about himself or herself. Some teenagers will develop great skill in deception to prevent people from being mad at them. Some will find comfort in overattaching to groups. Many will find ways of escaping their feelings by changing them with alcohol, drugs, nicotine, or other addictions. Adolescence is a very vulnerable time.

Teenagers will need to practice talking about feelings. It doesn't necessarily come naturally to them. The best way to help them is to talk to them about your own feelings. Tell your kids stories from your own teenage years and describe to them the emotions you faced and how you dealt with them.

Scott, age seventeen, recently was "dumped" by his girlfriend. His parents saw that he was really hurt, and his pain started to come out in angry ways. He was cruel to his younger brother and sister, was mad about homework, and didn't seem to want to go to any social or church activities. Scott's dad talked to him about a similar experience he had as a teenager.

"Scott, the same thing happened to me when I was seventeen. One day without warning, a girl I really cared about told me that she wanted to end our relationship. I was crushed, but I didn't want her or anyone else to know. So I acted cool, like it didn't bother me. I was really angry at all girls for a while. I took my anger out in a lot of inappropriate ways. In reality, though, I simply was sad. I missed her, but I was too 'tough' to cry. It was several years before I really got over my sadness. It took meeting and falling in love with your mother to restore my trust in girls again.

"I would suggest that you write a letter to your girlfriend that you will never send. Tell her how much you cared for her and how much you miss her. If you are angry with her for breaking up, tell her that in the letter too. And for right now, know that I love and support you. You're a handsome, talented, and great guy. Some girl will come along for you someday who will see that."

Several weeks later, Scott walked into his dad's study with tears in his eyes and showed him a letter he had written. His dad read it and hugged his son for a long time.

This story is great, and some teens have this kind of intimacy with their parents. But you may need to accept that part of the separation process involves individual identity formation, which means your teenagers may not want to talk to you about their intimate feelings. A child who has always been able to talk to you may now, as a teenager, become more silent around you or resist interacting. As hard as this will be on you, don't take this behavior as a sign of rejection, but as a normal part of the process of growing up. If you handle this with grace, your child will love you for it and be more able later, as an adult, to talk to you. Also, don't hesitate to welcome other safe adults into your teenager's life, people with whom he can practice sharing his feelings. I have always prayed for and been thankful for those pastors, teachers, and coaches who were able to fill this role for my children in a healthy way.

Depression

Symptoms of depression often signal unresolved emotional conflicts, but there can be medical reasons for depression also. It is wise to have a medical doctor or psychiatrist evaluate your child if he seems depressed, since some types of depression can be treated with medication. Even if medication is prescribed, psychological counseling may also be warranted. Below is a brief checklist of some symptoms of depression:

- mood swings: At times a teenager may seem very happy, but soon after seems extremely sad.
- loss of appetite: This is not necessarily about anorexia, but any severe weight loss should be checked out.
- disturbance of sleep: While it's normal for teenagers to sleep a lot, you should not avoid asking them about how they're feeling. An

inability to go to sleep could indicate anxiety which should definitely be investigated.

- bursts of anger: Volatility is a part of being a child. Temper tantrums are a symptom of being four, not necessarily of being a teenager.
- slipping grades: Otherwise good students suddenly, for no apparent reason (such as being in a sport or working long hours), start earning poor grades.
- loss of significant friendships: Again, for no clear reason, friends may disappear or change. If a teenager starts hanging out with other teenagers who seem troubled, this is not a good sign.
- drastic change in dress: Although teenagers may have weird dress habits influenced by passing fads, certain kinds of dress can signal danger. A current trend, for example, is called "gothic" or "Goth" in which teenagers wear black clothes and makeup. This may signify a preoccupation with darkness, evil, and even death. Closely identifying with people of similar dress may indicate participation in certain group cultic activities.
- addictive behavior: Smoking, drinking, or using other drugs can signal that teenagers are trying to medicate feelings of depression or anxiety. Simply telling them to stop won't work. Investigation must be made about what is going on.
- isolating: Seeking opportunities to be alone, such as always being in their room, can signal poor self-image and social skills, both of which definitely contribute to depression.

A teenager can be depressed for so many reasons, and it doesn't mean that you are a bad parent. But if you have done something to contribute to the problem, you can show courage by facing your mistakes and getting help for the entire family.

Talking to a depressed teen can be extremely frustrating. There is a fine balance between offering them love, support, and medical and psychological treatment, and challenging them to help themselves by dealing productively with their emotions. Some depression may be rooted in medical problems that teenagers can't resolve by themselves. Others may need to have tough discipline in their lives so they can make healthy decisions and take advantage of the emotional, spiritual, and medical help that is available. In dealing with depression, it is the rare parent who has the skill to figure out this balance alone. At times you will need help evaluating the situation and talking with your teen about what is going on. Getting that kind of professional help is not a sign of weakness in your family. It is a sign of strength.

Depressed kids are not able to complete some of the developmental tasks essential to healthy sexual development. Some teenagers, for instance, try to deal with depression by finding excitement or acceptance through sexual activity. Some symptoms of this might be changes in their attitudes about sex, being more sexual in their dress, using more sexual humor, having pornography in the home, forming new relationships with kids who seem to be sexually active, or participating in other sexual activity that you haven't known about before. Again, get help for your teenager's depression. You may also need to get help for any addictive sexual behaviors that have taken hold. One of the major challenges I face professionally is to provide adequate help and treatment for teenagers who have sexually addictive problems. If your teenager needs help, call the Oasis Ministry, a ministry that I direct, to get a referral in your area. See the resource section in this book for more information.

HEALTHY SEXUALITY DURING ADOLESCENCE: RELATIONAL DIMENSION

During puberty and early adolescence, children tend to look to relationships for selfish reasons. They are forming their own identities by attaching to others. As older adolescents, if they are maturing, they will seek relationships that are not so selfish. They will begin to learn the true meaning of friendship. This task can be confusing, as the quest for friendship is always mixed with the challenges of social, athletic, academic, and even spiritual competition. It is more likely, however, that they will find, maintain, and become better friends now that they are maturing.

Friendship

In chapter 2 we talked about the three Greek words for love: *eros, philia,* and *agape.* While the raging hormones of puberty that create raw sexual attraction *(eros)* have certainly not departed, now is the time to experiment with *philia,* the love of a brother or sister. It is much more common today for teenagers to have friends of the opposite sex who are not considered romantic or sexual partners. This is good. It is also more common for sex to take place between teenagers who have no true feelings of romantic attraction or love. This is not good. The result of this development is that sex has become more recreational.

In this stage conversations about sex must emphasize that men and women need to be friends before they are anything else. Dating and other forms of socializing should be for the purpose of developing friendships.

David and Heather had been dating for several weeks. They both felt sexual attraction for each other. David felt a rather urgent need to express that and tried to convince Heather that it was okay because they were such good friends and he really loved her. Heather responded that she loved him as a friend, but that sex was for a higher form of love, one to be found in marriage. David didn't understand that, but Heather's friendship was important to him, so he decided to honor her boundary.

I wish that all dating situations worked out like that. Unfortunately, as we all know, they don't. You will have to remind your teenagers that, if they are to honor their commitment to save sex until marriage, they may lose some friends along the way. David and Heather's response to sexual pressure indicates that they have developed in a very important way. Heather was secure enough in her own self to be able to make a healthy decision. She risked losing David, but that was a risk she was willing to take. She wasn't so dependent on David that she went along with his demands. David valued friendship above sex. He didn't need sex to be a sign to him that Heather loved him.

Sexual Abstinence

During the teenage years the primary sexual issue for your child is to make a personal decision to abstain from sex until marriage. Organizations such as "True Love Waits" provide literature about formalizing this decision. It is not unlike the decision to accept Christ. This should be a formal and celebrated decision, not just something that is taken for granted because a teenager is a Christian. Organizations that support teens who make this decision also provide the accountability of groups of like-minded peers. This kind of peer support can't be underestimated. In our current culture it is vital.

The most important thing parents can do during this stage is to help their teens develop a vision for marital sexuality that is worth waiting for. It is one thing to know the possible painful emotional, physical, and spiritual consequences of premarital sexuality. It is a more effective strategy to create a vision of the true goal: the intimate marriage, faithfulness to one person for life. I will say more about this in the spiritual dimension, but I believe that it is partly the job of married couples to testify to the validity and beauty of this vision. If your church doesn't provide this kind of resource to the teenagers, encourage your pastor to consider it. Better yet, volunteer to head up a task force in your church that will actively work to support teens in a commitment to sexual abstinence.

Dating

The age at which kids start to date varies. Parents have different ideas about when dating becomes appropriate. The key issue is determining at what stage teenagers are mature enough to make appropriate decisions. There is no arbitrary starting point that is right for everyone. As you assess your teenager's maturity and ability to make healthy decisions, your job is to set boundaries that will help keep dating situations as safe as possible. This includes enforcing reasonable curfews, making sure teens are not entertaining each other when parents aren't home, monitoring phone privileges, and knowing your child's whereabouts.

The idea of a conventional date, at least in the sense that many of us experienced it, is less popular today. It is now more common for kids to gather in groups. Parents will need to set boundaries concerning how many kids are allowed over, how late they can stay, whether or not smoking is allowed outside (or inside), and what the rules are regarding alcohol. Teenagers will want to participate in "sleepovers" so that they can stay up late and be together. This is another scenario about which you will want to set boundaries. I know of some parents who have permitted coed sleepovers. I'm sure their kids have assured them that no smoking, drinking, or sex goes on at this kind of gathering and that everyone is just friends. My feeling is that such an unscheduled and spontaneous gathering is a problem waiting to happen. You must make careful, conscious decisions about how much of this you will allow.

Jenny, sixteen, was part of a group that enjoyed being together. She liked Dick, one of the boys in this group. This group liked to go to one another's houses. They often started an evening without quite knowing where they would end up. Sometimes they went from house to house. Toward the end of the evening, boys and girls would pair off and be with each other, occasionally for various levels of sexual activity. Many of these kids smoked. It seemed that alcohol was always around.

Jenny and Dick had paired off a number of times. They had "made out" on these occasions, but it hadn't gotten too involved. Dick began drinking more and more at these gatherings. One night, while drunk, he became more sexually aggressive than ever before. Jenny said no, but Dick didn't seem to want to stop. Eventually one of the other girls came into the room and intervened.

When Jenny got home, she was an emotional wreck. Her mother discovered her

*in her room crying. After she found out what was going on and that Jenny was phys-
ically all right, she said, "That must have been really frightening. Tell me about it."
Jenny talked and talked. Then she asked her mom, "What did I do wrong? Dick was
never like that before."*

*Her mom said, "There is absolutely nothing you did that justified Dick being sex-
ually forceful with you. He was completely wrong, and I'm so sorry about what happened to you. Alcohol will sometimes tear down a person's inhibitions, allowing him
or her to give in to their drives and impulses. This is what happened to Dick. This was
about Dick and not about you."*

*Later, Jenny and her mom continued to talk. Her mom asked, "Do you think that
this is the kind of boy you want to be around? You know, I think that you need to make
some decisions about this group. There are many nice kids in it, and I know that you
have really liked Dick. But sometimes people in groups follow the example of what the
group is doing. If you spend time around people who are smoking and drinking, bad
things can happen."*

This is a supportive and loving mom. What happened to Jenny could
have escalated into a date rape had her friend not intervened. Jenny will need
to talk about her fears some more. Jenny's mom and dad may need to help
her make decisions about who she hangs around with.

Community

Teenagers who don't have specific activities to focus on may get bored
and restless and do destructive things. One of the more proactive things
parents can do is to encourage their teenagers to be involved in church, social,
and athletic activities that have meaning in people's lives. It might be a youth
group, a school club, a service organization, or a team sport. Teenagers need
a community of friends in which to belong and to find purpose.

*Tony, age sixteen, was like many kids his age. He didn't seem to have a lot going
on in his life that was worthwhile or even interesting to him. He had stopped playing*

a couple of sports he'd previously been involved in because he'd been cut from the teams. He was restless and bored. He tended to stay out late with his friends and sleep late in the morning when he didn't have to go to school. He went to youth group on Sunday mornings, but he didn't like participating in the social activities during the week.

Tony's parents sat him down one day and presented him with a decision. "We love you and hate to see you without something meaningful to look forward to. We have a list of various activities available to you at school, in the community, and at church. We want you to pick one of the church activities and one other activity to try. You can decide what appeals to you the most, but we feel strongly that this is something you need to do."

Tony may balk at his parents' direction, but this may be one of their last opportunities to directly influence his choices in regard to relationships. To simply allow him to float through these years with no sense of community or meaning is to abandon him when he needs them most. Kids who experience community and a sense of belonging develop stronger friendships. They are more confident and self-assured. They are less vulnerable to the temptations connected with dangerous relationships and meaninglessness in their lives.

HEALTHY SEXUALITY DURING ADOLESCENCE: PERSONAL DIMENSION

Remember, this dimension is about preventing and healing psychosexual wounds and about the healthy development of sexual identity and self-perception. The issues described in the personal dimension of the last chapter may not be resolved at this age, so more work may need to be done. Development of personal integrity and maturity depends on healthy resolution of earlier issues.

Shame and Control Issues

As we discussed in the physical dimension, losing weight, gaining weight, looking sexy, and building muscles are examples of what teens may do to gain a sense of control. A key issue to consider is what thoughts and feelings would cause them to take such great pains to control their appearance. Shame is often at the root of control, and sometimes it goes much deeper and is more personal than the kind of generalized shame inflicted by our beauty-obsessed culture.

Tammy was sexually molested by her brother when she was small. Her parents found out about her brother's behavior and put an abrupt halt to it, but they wrongly assumed that Tammy wasn't damaged by the experience. No one in the family ever talked about it again. As she developed, Tammy lived in fear that men would find her irresistibly attractive. She discovered that she got much less male attention when she gained enough weight to camouflage her figure.

Tammy is like thousands of people who think they can control other people's reactions by how they look. In this case, Tammy is trying to control men's reactions to her because of the fear created by sexual trauma. Fortunately, her parents started putting two and two together as they watched their lovely daughter get bigger and bigger during her teenage years. Being very careful not to shame her for her appearance or eating habits, they sat down with her one weekend and had a discussion about the sexual trauma she had experienced and how they suspected it was affecting her development now. This discussion opened the door to many more, and eventually the entire family got some counseling to address the complex problems created by unresolved sexual abuse.

Another way that an adolescent's sexual shame and pain may express itself is through sexually acting out.

Bonnie became sexually involved with several older boys in her neighborhood when she was seven. It seemed like sexual play or experimentation, but "playing" like this with more sexually developed boys was very damaging to Bonnie. Her father worked hard and wasn't home as much as he would have liked. These older boys gave Bonnie lots of attention and seemed to want to be with her. When Bonnie's parents discovered what was happening, they took steps to shield her from further experiences like this.

Since she was somewhat shy and isolated as an adolescent, Bonnie's parents were really surprised when, at age seventeen, she began dressing provocatively. She started dating a boy they didn't approve of. While they were trying to figure out what to do and how to get at the root of Bonnie's behavior, she was headed for trouble.

Bonnie had learned a message about sex ten years earlier: If you want male attention, you get it sexually. She was playing out that message in her teenage years. She was also buying into the lie that sex equals love. If teenagers feel that the only way to know they are lovable is to be sexual, they may begin a pursuit of sex that can lead to unhealthy relationships, and even to sexual addiction.

Bonnie's parents didn't know all the reasons for her behavior, but they sat down with her one day, and her father opened a discussion that led to a lot of healing in the months ahead.

"Bonnie, I've noticed that you've been wearing clothes that really send out a sexual message. You are a beautiful young woman, and many boys and men will respond to that message for all the wrong reasons. When you were young, the things that those older boys did to you were wrong. You didn't deserve for them to happen. It wasn't about anything that you said or did. I know that I wasn't around for you enough back then. I'm really sorry. It wasn't because I didn't love you. I was trying to work hard and provide for the family. It was wrong not to give you more time. I'm going to try to correct that, and I hope that it is not too late. Most of all you need to know that you have a wonderful mind and spirit. I hope that some young man will take the time to get to know you, to love you for who you are, not just for what you look like."

Bonnie's dad had to repeat this loving message many times and honor his commitment to spend more time with his daughter. She also got some professional counseling so she could talk through her earlier life experiences and understand the powerful impact they had had on her self-perception and her approach to relationships.

Parents need to be aware that one of the reasons teenagers can be anxious, depressed, or shame-bound is that they are dealing with unresolved trauma. They have been physically, emotionally, sexually, or spiritually invaded or abandoned. The result is that they feel like "bad" people. Their logic is simple: Good things happen to good people, bad things happen to bad people. One of the symptoms of unresolved trauma is how they are currently experiencing relationships and their own sexuality. You will want to monitor your children closely on these issues.

Homosexuality

In the last chapter I covered some major points about homosexuality. A same-sex orientation usually begins to become apparent, at least in a the privacy of a child's mind, during puberty. During the teenage years, a child who believes he or she is homosexual usually will experience increasingly intense feelings of confusion, shame, fear, and despair. This is especially true if he has been raised in the church, where homosexuality is rarely accepted and most often is heatedly condemned. Many gay teenagers attempt or commit suicide.

Suspecting that their child is struggling with homosexuality usually produces great fear, uncertainty, and often anger in parents. What should they do? Is it their fault? What will people think? What does God think? When parents are consumed with fear, shame, and self-doubt, it is almost impossible for them to effectively converse with their child about his sexuality. Many parents react in a way that only increases their child's despair, which often only drives him farther away from getting the understanding and help he needs.

If you suspect your child is attracted to the same sex or if he comes to you and says he is gay, I encourage you to remember two major points.

First, people become homosexually oriented for a variety of reasons. A healthy parent will be open to any contribution he or she has made and is willing to try to correct it. It never helps the current situation to beat yourself up. You simply don't know what factors have created this situation. It may have nothing to do with you at all. There is still a lot of uncertainty about the myriad causes of homosexuality. We have some good ideas, but any person who believes that he or she is gay will represent a complex interaction of factors. Better to work for a solution with caring professionals who can help untangle these factors than to feel so desperately guilty that you become immobilized.

Second, it never helps to be angry at your child. Remember that people who feel they are homosexual don't think they have made a conscious choice to be this way. Most of them have honestly struggled with feeling different and have asked "Why?" Many have prayed to be different and have emotionally battled their orientation for years. Many have been afraid that if they tell anyone they will be ridiculed, rejected, or ostracized. The worst thing that can happen to them is to experience rejection from their parents. You need to enter the struggle with them, hear the pain, seek to be supportive, and offer to find help.

If you are facing this situation, one of the worst things you can do is to expect your child to understand your emotions about his orientation. You can't talk a child out of homosexuality by telling him how much he has hurt you. Don't be dramatically hysterical, pained, and a victim. Don't expect your child to resolve your sadness or guilt. Instead, find support from adults who can listen and pray with you. If possible, find other parents who have lived through this experience.

Some people who believe they are gay have been reoriented to heterosexuality through intense psychotherapy and spiritual healing. By the teenage years, however, this healing can be a painfully long process, one that involves years of counseling. If some form of trauma is a factor, that pain alone will take time to heal. Be available to face that journey with your child in the most supportive way you can.

The bottom line is simple: State your beliefs to your teenager and offer to find professional help for him if he is willing to explore the complex issues involved in his orientation. If he rejects all offers of help, then you have a choice. Before you make this decision, pray, pray, and then pray some more. The first option is to let him go in love, as did the father of the prodigal in Jesus' parable, hoping that one day he will seek help. I have known this to happen many times. The other option is to intervene as you would with an alcoholic. An intervention involves stating your beliefs about the behavior and outlining consequences if help is not sought. In my opinion this approach is risky because it reinforces a gay person's belief that he is being victimized, which may only drive him deeper into rebellion. The single most important thing you can do for your homosexual child is to love him, love him, love him.

Here is what one loving father I know told his son:

"Son, I hear what you're telling Mom and me. You feel that you are gay. Thank you for having the courage to tell us. I know that this must have been a real struggle for you. First, I want you to know that I love you. I may not have been very good about telling you that or demonstrating it to you. I'm telling you now. I love you. At the same time, I feel that it is against God's design for you to sexually act out in a homosexual way. This is not because God doesn't understand and simply wants to punish you. He knows how you have struggled with this and will always be there for you whether you believe it or not. You may even be angry at God, thinking that he made you this way or that he won't change you. But God loves you in more wonderful ways than I ever could. Nevertheless, I believe the Bible teaches that homosexuality is wrong, and I think that's because God is pointing us to the highest possible relationship, that 'one-flesh' union between a man and woman.

"If you are ever going to experience that, you will need lots of guidance and support. Mom and I will do whatever we can to see that you get that. I understand that many gay people believe they are born the way they are. I'm willing to be wrong, but I don't think that is true. I believe emotional forces inside you—forces you're not even aware of—pushed you in this direction.

"Most of all, I want you to know that I understand how lonely this struggle must have been for you. I'm really sad that you haven't been able to talk with me about it before, but I understand how frightened you must have been about what I would think. Please know, Son, that there is nothing you could ever do that would stop me from loving you. I can only imagine and not really comprehend what this must have been like for you. I find myself wondering if your quest is not really about finding love and nurture from other men. Men are not too good at finding that in each other. I accept that you need the touch, warmth, and understanding of other men. Believe it or not, I do too. But being sexual with them is not the deepest form of getting that.

"I would also encourage you to allow your spirit to find deep friendship with other women. In a way, not feeling sexual toward them is a deeply freeing experience that allows you to enjoy the emotional and spiritual nature of friendship between a man and woman. I believe that many women out there would love you in deeply caring ways even if they knew the truth about what you struggle with."

This father has done the right thing. He is probably angry and frightened himself, but he is choosing not to show this anger and fear to his son. This is the loving thing to do. The son needs support, and he needs to be pointed in the right direction.

The argument about the "nature versus nurture" origin of homosexuality may never be settled scientifically. How to deal with the whole issue is going to be an ongoing struggle between various groups of people who are ostensibly trying to do the loving thing. My prayer is that the children and teenagers who are hurting and need parental support don't get lost in the middle of the struggle.

Aberrant Behavior

The term *aberrant* means behavior that deviates from the norm. Most cultures try to define normal. Certainly, the Bible does. Our culture and the Bible are often at odds when it comes to defining what is sexually normal, but in this section I would like to consider sexual behavior that even society would consider abnormal. This is a very painful subject because the behaviors that I am going to mention are completely disgusting to most people. They are, however, more common than most people realize. My motivation for including this section is my professional experience that convinces me that most of these kind of behaviors start in adolescence. Teenagers who are involved in aberrant sexual behaviors usually think that they are the only ones doing them and will feel tremendous shame. This shame drives them further into silence. When shame perpetuates silence, behaviors like these fester and can become very destructive.

I am going to mention only a handful of these behaviors in several broad categories. Within each category are variations so plentiful that psychologists have catalogued more than four hundred specific behaviors within just one of the categories. When you read this section and you have a sense of something demonic, you are right.

Fetishes. A fetish is the use of an object or ritualized behavior to enhance sexual excitement, either during masturbation or sexual intercourse.

Gary's mom was putting underwear away in his drawer one day and found a number of girl's undergarments inside. At first she thought that maybe these were "souvenirs" of his sexual experience with girls. This, by itself, shocked her. Gary's parents talked to him about this discovery. Among other concerns, they were worried he might get some girl pregnant. Very painfully, Gary said, "I've never had intercourse with a girl. Those are things I use when I masturbate."

In Gary's case, underwear is the fetish. Any object or repeated behavior can work. One of the fetishes that has killed many teenagers is masturbating while using something to almost strangle oneself. The experience of the diminished air supply to the brain heightens the pleasure of orgasm. The key to understanding fetishes is to look past the pure lust and determine the symbolic nature of the object or activity. Female underwear in this case is directly symbolic of female presence and nurture. It is safe to say that Gary is a lonely boy looking for female nurture. His quest for this has become associated with sex. He will have to get professional help to "unhook" this connection.

When Peter was small, his mother was taught that a child needs to have regular bowel movements and that it may be necessary to use enemas to achieve this. For years she would give him these. Later, in his teenage years, Peter inserted various things into his rectum during masturbation. Still later, in marriage, he talked his wife into doing this.

Again, Peter's case is not hard to figure out. In his sexual life he was re-creating his experience with his mother. Although the original circumstances were extremely embarrassing, he wanted to bring back the sense of closeness he felt at that time.

Voyeurism. This involves looking at someone else, uninvited, for the purpose of sexual excitement. Some people may go around neighborhoods looking into windows, but voyeurism begun in adolescence is much more common and varied than this.

When Russell was seventeen, he found himself drawn to the window of his neighbor's house. He would go there when the women in that house were bathing. He felt shameful, but it was really exciting.

Many of you recognize this kind of story. After all, it is not uncommon for children of all ages to want to "see" what the opposite sex is like. At age seventeen, however, this curiosity has been mixed with sexual excitement and may lead to more serious and intrusive behaviors if help is not found.

Like most activities mentioned in this section, voyeurism is a lonely quest to see something that one thinks he can't possess. A young man looking at his naked mother or sisters is trying to feel close to their femaleness. The main thing to remember is that, while voyeurism is about sexual excitement, it is more deeply about a longing for female nurture. Understanding parents will help their children understand this and help them meet this need in a loving way.

Exhibitionism. As with voyeurism, we have stereotypes of the old man in the raincoat exposing himself. Teenagers can be much more creative.

Mary, age eighteen, enjoyed being a woman and getting the attention of men. In the last several months, she had discovered that she attracted a lot of attention when she didn't wear a bra. She got more daring with this. One night, she decided to wear a blouse that was fairly sheer. When she went out with her friends, who seemed embarrassed by her attire, she reveled in the stares that men gave her.

Brad, age sixteen, liked to leave his bedroom door open, particularly when his sisters were around. He would wait for them to pass by and pretend to be getting dressed. He enjoyed their surprised reactions. When he went to the mall, he also liked to try on clothes and leave the dressing room door open, trying to spark a similar reaction from women in the store. Since he began driving, he has been trying to expose himself to women who drive by in vans and are sitting high enough to see down into his car.

Both Brad's and Mary's situations are getting worse and may require intervention. Brad's most recent behavior may even cause him to get arrested. Many parents I know who have faced these situations hope that it is a one-time occurrence and that the problem will go away. But I urge you to take it seriously. Exhibitionism means something. You may notice that both Brad and Mary seek the attention that they are getting. Their actions are not just about sex but about needing attention. If you ignore such behavior, it may only get worse.

Inappropriate touch. This occurs when someone touches someone else and gets a sense of sexual excitement from it. The person being touched may not even be aware of it.

Phil, age nineteen, had to ride the bus to college every day. He enjoyed it when the bus got crowded. He would try to position himself close to attractive girls or women. Simply being that close to them gave him pleasurable sexual feelings. He learned that he could occasionally get away with touching them, and they wouldn't get mad. One woman even seemed to enjoy it and invited him over to her apartment.

Phil is on a downward spiral. If he doesn't get help, he may go on to more serious behavior that is more aggressive in nature. Like the others in this section, he is looking for attention and a reaction mixed with the sexual high of the experience.

Phone sex. This involves seeking a sexual high from talking about sex or being sexual over the phone. These days, a number of phone-sex services even advertise in the local newspaper. They offer sexual conversation for a price.

Dave's parents were shocked when they got their monthly phone bill. It was over $500. Almost all of the calls were to a number with a 900 prefix. When Dave's dad called this number, a very sensuous female voice welcomed him and asked what kind of woman he would like to talk to.

The way these phone companies advertise suggests their appeal. Their "service" is supposedly only about sex, but one of the ads said, "Are you lonely tonight?" Teenagers who get involved in these kind of activities may feel lonely and socially out of it; they may believe they have no friends—certainly no real friends of the opposite sex.

Ann felt herself continually drawn to her father's computer. She had discovered the "chat rooms" available there. She found several men who seemed really nice, and she developed relationships with them. Ann was tempted to give one of them her phone number so they could talk on the phone.

Every day thousands of teenagers visit Internet chat rooms. It is a growing epidemic. In chat rooms you'll find people masquerading under false identities so they can prey on young people and teenagers. Those who get drawn in are often lonely and need help.

Bestiality. This is sex with animals. In many other parts of the world, an entire segment of pornography is dedicated to this activity. Such behavior is very common among teenagers. Sex with dogs or farm animals is not just a rural phenomenon. I have known many teenagers who became sexual with the family pet. When you think about it, a pet is loyal and faithful, always there, and attentive. You see the connection with emotional needs and sexual excitement.

Pain exchange. This is the sexual excitement that occurs for some people when they either receive or inflict pain.

Beth was molested by her uncle and older brothers when she was five. She told her mother, who was so angry she first slapped her and then spanked her and told her never to talk about it again. The molestation continued, and whenever she brought it up Beth would be slapped or spanked. When she turned eighteen, she got involved with a boy who was angry and liked to slap her. More and more throughout her life, she allowed herself to get involved in relationships in which pain was a part of sex.

You see here a behavior that is the result of serious trauma for Beth. For her, healing began when she was able to go past addressing the sexual sin and start dealing with the incest and abuse.

Prostitution. Sadly, more teenagers, both male and female, get involved each year in trading sex for money. They are feeling lonely, depressed, unloved, and perhaps desperate for money. They find adults who seem to care and love them but who wind up using the teens in this way for their own gain. I have been surprised over the years at how many former prostitutes I've counseled come from fairly prosperous, sometimes even Christian, families. Somewhere in their lives, they learned that they can use their bodies to get money and what they think is love, attention, and even a sense of power over those they become involved with.

Transgender behavior. This kind of acting out involves confusion about one's identity as a male or female. It is different from homosexuality. Homosexuals have sexual attraction to the same sex. Transgendered individuals believe that they are females born into a male body or vice versa. It is estimated that several thousand sex-change operations are performed in this country every year. This is the adult result of this confusion.

All of these adults trace their feelings back to childhood. You will remember that in the first three years of life, all kids have those questions about whether they are boys or girls. For some, this confusion lasts into adult years.

If you have an open and honest relationship with your child, he or she may be able to tell you about feelings like these. But because complex early emotional issues are involved, professional help will be needed if this confusion persists into adolescence. One sign of this confusion is cross-dressing behavior, but it's necessarily prompted by the same reasons.

Cross-dressing, or transvestism. Cross-dressing is dressing in the clothes of the opposite sex. Many cross-dressers function in heterosexual marriages. Cross-dressing is not necessarily related to homosexuality.

Cross-dressing may also be called transvestism. This is confusing because there is a distinction. Cross-dressers may not completely assume the identity of a person of the opposite sex like a transvestite does. A transvestite not only cross-dresses, but will try to effect in every way the appearance of the opposite sex. There are complicated reasons for this, and either condition requires professional help.

Aaron, age three, had a mom who had always wanted a girl but never had one. So she treated Aaron like a girl most of the time. She even occasionally dressed him in girl's clothing. In his teen years, Aaron found himself still stealing his mother's clothes and dressing like a woman. He found it sexually exciting. He dated and eventually got married, but continued to find sexual excitement when he wore his wife's clothing. He even liked going shopping with her for clothes and tried to get her to participate in his fantasies.

This story underscores the reality that a child learns a great deal about gender identity from his or her parents. It also suggests that Aaron's mom probably had an indication of the problem he was having in adolescence when some of her clothes disappeared. Do you see the denial that some parents choose because of their own guilt and shame about how they may have contributed to their child's problem?

Incest. This is sex between biologically related members of a family. For many people, the perpetrator of their sexual abuse was an older brother or sister. If you are facing this serious situation, you will need to get professional help for the whole family. Don't panic. Incest does not mean that you have a bad family or that someone is going to get hauled off by government authorities. Competent professionals can lead your children and the entire family through a healing process.

I know many families who don't confront the situation and who harbor the secret all of their lives. So often brothers and sisters won't talk to each other, their marriages are troubled, and the legacy of the abuse is passed down to future generations.

Now take a deep breath, and remember God's grace and sovereign power. God is in control and can heal any of these situations if they are brought to him. All of the stories and examples in this section, as in this entire book, are based on the experiences of real people. They should alert you to Satan's great power to deceive and of the great lengths he will go to destroy a life. As parents, you need to take seriously any behavior you discover that is abnormal. Let me also remind you, however, that God's power is stronger than Satan's. All of the people in these stories are now adults in the process of embracing healing, restoring marriages, and living Christ-centered lives.

You may have noticed that in this last section I did not include conversations between parent and child. Each of these situations requires specialized treatment, and it is best to leave much of that to professionals. You can, however, say some general things to your beloved child if you discover that he or she is participating in any of these aberrant behaviors:

- "I love you."
- "These behaviors make us angry, but we are not angry with you."
- "God still loves you."
- "We will walk with you during any consequences that you may experience."
- "We will help you make restitution for any wrongs you have committed."
- "You may think that you are the only one doing these things, but there are many others. Paul said in 1 Corinthians 10:13 that there is no temptation (sexual or otherwise) that is not common to man."
- "You may feel that you were born with these problems, but you were not. You can live a moral and pure life."
- "I/we will get you the help that you need."
- "Whatever I/we have done to contribute to your struggles, we are sorry and are willing to be a part of the healing process with you."
- "If you are angry with us, please know that we will listen and try to understand."
- "You may have been tempted to take your own life because of these things. Is that true? If so, we will get you help immediately. You are extremely precious to us and to God."

HEALTHY SEXUALITY DURING ADOLESCENCE: SPIRITUAL DIMENSION

During a teenager's process of individuation, she may question truths that she earlier accepted at face value. Unlike younger children, teenagers won't believe something simply because someone else told them to or because they belong to a certain group. This may discourage you, but please understand that it is a normal part of the maturing process. As parents you need to encourage your teenagers to think for themselves and then allow that to happen. If you push your own beliefs too hard and give them no room to question and explore, then they may rebel. As always, they will respond to positive role models rather than negative warnings and commands.

Creating a Vision for Purity

Most teenagers go through periods when they question God's design for sex: "Why should we wait, particularly when the whole world seems to be enjoying sex?"

It is a legitimate question. God has a higher calling for sex that what our culture offers. In a way we are asking teenagers to take a risk that God's calling truly is better. We are asking them to resist their natural biological longings in order to wait for the fulfillment of a higher spiritual experience.

God's design for sex is for our benefit, not to repress us or leave us feeling left out. This truth can be hard for adolescents to grasp or appreciate. This is where our own past experience as adolescents and young adults can play a powerful teaching role. Our teenagers aren't particularly interested in hearing us pontificate about rules and morals, but they are more likely to listen to our honest expression of joy and pain as it relates to our own past decisions to remain abstinent or to be sexual before marriage. Sometimes sharing our own failures and successes is the most effective way to teach our kids what we want them to know. Rather than simply asking our children for a commitment to abstinence, we can help stoke their vision for purity and marital fidelity.

Harry took his son David, age seventeen, out for lunch one day. He empathized with him about what a crazy world it is out there sexually. Then he told a story from his own adolescence. "When I was your age, I was in love with a girl. We had been dating for a year. One night we went ahead and had sex, and it happened several more times. Then we went off to college and drifted apart. When I was in college, I met your mom. She knows about this, and she knew before we were married. She has forgiven me and we have a great relationship, but I have always regretted not waiting for your mom. I know that God has forgiven me, and I accept that. It's like other mistakes we make in life: As we look back, we wish it had been different. I'm simply trying to challenge you, if possible, to learn from my mistake and not make the same one."

By sharing personal experiences and telling stories, parents are more likely to get through to their teenagers about the spiritual value of remaining celibate until marriage. It's not just about following the rules; it's about the highest form of love, *agape* love.

In Matthew 5:17 Jesus addressed those who questioned his authority and his teaching: "Do not think that I have come to abolish the Law or the Prophets; I have not come to abolish them but to fulfill them." Jesus was continually being challenged by the chief priests, scribes, and Pharisees. They protected the law in a rather rigid and adolescent fashion. It was more important to them to obey the law than to understand why they were doing it. Jesus told them that there is a higher truth behind God's law, and Jesus himself came to fulfill it by pouring out his life for the love of humankind.

It is so important that parents teach their teenagers about *agape* love and how it relates to sexuality. In Matthew 22:37-40, Jesus said that the two greatest commandments are to love God and to love your neighbor as yourself. Sexual faithfulness in marriage is the fulfillment of true love between husband and wife. This is the spiritual reason behind our encouragement that our kids wait until they're married to have sex.

Perhaps you are divorced from your child's other parent and are currently single or remarried. Ever since your divorce, you have been explaining to your children that it wasn't about your love for them. Hopefully, you have cooperated as best you can with your former spouse to coordinate the healthy nurturing of your child. Now is not a bad time to have a conversation with your child about why the divorce happened and reaffirm your belief in the sanctity of marriage. You will undoubtedly face some of your own shame about this. Be gentle with yourself. God's grace is for you. You did what you felt was best and what may have been the safest at the time.

Explain this to your child while at the same time affirming the possibility of a wonderful marriage for yourself and for your child.

Mary's mom and dad divorced when she was eleven. Mary's dad had an affair and wasn't willing to give it up, so he filed for divorce. Mary's mom has had several conversations with her like this one:

"Mary, we have talked many times about how both your dad and I love you very much, even though we are no longer married. We are really sorry that our marriage didn't make it. Your dad has talked to you about what was going on with him. I don't know if he has ever apologized to you, but I want to now. It takes two people to make a marriage work, and we weren't able to do that. It's not my job to blame your dad. You know about what happened at the time. That is between your dad and God. I'm really sorry that we couldn't stay together for you. That was my goal, but it just didn't work.

"I do want you to know that I believe in marriage. It can be a wonderful thing. Millions of people stay sexually faithful to each other. Many marriages are shaken by infidelity, but the couple is able to work things out. Your dad and I didn't find a way to resolve all these issues, but that doesn't mean other people can't, with God's help. God intends for two people to be together for a lifetime. In that context, I believe that sex can be a beautiful and fulfilling thing. Your dad and I had some unhealed wounds from our childhood that made sex hard for us. We could have worked that out, but we didn't.

"You need to make your own decisions. There are many wonderful men out there who will love you completely. You have become a beautiful woman. I am so proud of you, and I pray for you every day."

This mother seems healed of her grief and anger over the divorce. But even if she hasn't fully recovered, she has chosen to affirm the vision and value of a healthy marriage. What a wonderful gift to her teenage daughter!

To give our teenagers a vision for purity, we need to have many conversations with them about spiritual principles and biblical values. One of the tasks for adolescents as they mature is to understand the character of God and how who he is relates to who they are becoming. God gives us rules that are good for us, but sometimes they feel painful or restrictive. A teenager who is learning to trust in the goodness of God and the reliability of God's wisdom will be more likely to wrestle deeply and productively with the spiritual implications of sexuality and sexual behavior.

The Power of God

A teenager who believes he has personal access to the power of God will also be more likely to explore the ways in which God can sustain him during temptation and protect him from sin.

One of my favorite stories in Scripture is in Numbers 13 and 14. I'd encourage you to read these two chapters. Moses was trying to prepare the Jews to enter the Promised Land. He sent out twelve spies, one from each of the twelve tribes, to scout things out. When they came back with a report, ten of them were really scared. They said that the land was exceedingly good, but that there were many obstacles, like giants. They even said, "We seemed like grasshoppers...to them." (Numbers 13:33). In other words, "There is no way we're going there!"

The crowd of Jewish people was really depressed and disappointed by this news. They were infected with negative thinking. One of the other spies, Caleb, tried to quiet the crowd and give them confidence, but they wouldn't listen. They cried out with passion, "If only we had died in Egypt! Or in this desert!" (Numbers 14:2). Even Moses and his brother Aaron fell on their faces in despair.

Then Joshua, the leader for the next generation, stepped forward. He expressed his confidence in God's power, "If the LORD is pleased with us, he will lead us into that land...and will give it to us" (Numbers 14:8).

This story doesn't deal overtly with sexuality, but it reminds us that any goal worth attaining may seem impossible on the front end. To draw an analogy, we could think of the vision of attaining fidelity in marriage or maintaining abstinence as a single person as the Promised Land. It is God's plan for our lives. It is where he wants us to go. It is an experience flowing with milk and honey. Young people today face "giant" obstacles as they attempt to enter the Promised Land. You will notice that the pessimism of the ten reluctant spies was contagious. Caleb was the first to suggest that success was possible. He had confidence, but that by itself was not enough. The people grumbled. To them it seemed wiser to return to Egypt, where they at least knew what to expect. The people who had been wandering in the desert for years preferred go back to slavery and die.

In many ways, our current culture is like a desert. Sexual lust, perversion, and emptiness is slavery. To aspire to something higher, something that God promises, will require facing giant cultural influences. Young Joshua, the leader for the next generation, not only had confidence, he had trust. He said that the people could enter the Promised Land with God's help. This is the message that we must instill in young people today. There is a higher calling that at times will seem impossible to reach. It is not better, however, to go back to the slavery of sexual sin. It is better to have a confident vision and to trust God to help us get to the land flowing with milk and honey.

When any of us aspire to this higher vision, we will seem like "grasshoppers" to those around us. We will seem different, old-fashioned, repressed, and intolerant. Our spiritual battle, as Paul said, is not against human tribes such as the Jews faced; it is against principalities and powers, the devil himself. But we can win the fight with God's help.

> Finally, be strong in the Lord and in his mighty power. Put on the full armor of God so that you can take your stand against the devil's schemes. For our struggle is not against flesh and blood, but against the rulers, against the authorities, against the powers of this dark world and against the spiritual forces of evil in the heavenly realms. Therefore put on the full armor of God, so that when the day of evil comes, you may be able to stand your ground, and after you have done everything, to stand. Stand firm then, with the belt of truth buckled around your waist, with the breastplate of righteousness in place, and with your feet fitted

with the readiness that comes from the gospel of peace. In addition to all this, take up the shield of faith, with which you can extinguish all the flaming arrows of the evil one. Take the helmet of salvation and the sword of the Spirit, which is the word of God. And pray in the Spirit on all occasions with all kinds of prayers and requests. With this in mind, be alert and always keep on praying for all the saints. (Ephesians 6:10-18)

Young people will need to arm themselves for the fight. As warriors, they will need to have a vision of what they are fighting for as well as the spiritual armor and weapons to achieve victory over the Evil One.

Sometimes kids will not readily understand why they need this vision or why God's protection is necessary. Following is a true story that I have used to try to explain to teenagers why certain restrictions and protections are in their best interest, even when they are hard to understand.

When Chris was eighteen months old, he was eating a peanut. His brother came up behind him and startled him, causing Chris to gasp. As he did, peanut fragments got sucked into his lungs and blocked his airway. The next day his mom noticed that he was having trouble breathing. His parents rushed Chris to the hospital, where an x-ray revealed that his right lung had collapsed. Emergency surgery removed the peanut fragments, and the lung filled back up. The doctor said that Chris was lucky; he had been about thirty minutes away from dying.

Chris had to be in the intensive care unit for a while. Before he woke up from the anesthesia, he lay there bound to the bed so that he wouldn't accidentally yank the IV needles out of his arm or the oxygen mask off his face. His dad stood by his bed as he woke up, opened his eyes, and realized the scary place he was in and the pain he felt. He lifted up his little arms with the IVs in him and cried, "Dad!"

The father knew that he couldn't pick him up, that he needed to be in this restricted bed, and that the oxygen was life-giving. He had no way to explain this to his young son. He put his hand on Chris, told him he loved him over and over again, and tried to calm him the best he could.

I believe that this father's experience illustrates how God sometimes feels as he deals with us. We don't have the maturity, experience, or ability to communicate with him or to understand why certain things are the way they are. But God knows that his life-giving restrictions are the very stuff of spiritual breathing. Sexual purity is like this. Teenagers may not fully understand why they should say no to certain things, other than to please God, until they experience the nature of *agape* love with their spouse. Meanwhile, it's the job of parents to continue setting boundaries, presenting truth, and explaining the spiritual value of sexual abstinence.

The Grace of God

I have referred to my own sexual sins of the past. When I finally became broken and repentant about those, went to get help, and began a journey of healing for myself and my wife, for the first time I began to experience and appreciate the grace of God.

At some point, my wife and I knew that we had to explain to our kids about all the tears and the many hours spent away from them in counseling and support groups. We also knew that our own relationship had not been the best model of a healthy couple or healthy parents. We had done many things that might have wounded them in some way.

At the time our kids were five, eight, and eleven. One night we sat them down and began explaining to them what had been going on. I told them the general nature of my sins. We talked to them about what we had been doing to heal as individuals and as a couple. We assured them over and over again that we were going to stay married and that they didn't have to worry. Finally, we said, "We know that in all of this we haven't always been the best parents. You have seen us fight or be distant. We haven't always been there for you. There have been times when we were so sad or frightened that you must have worried about us. We're sorry for the ways we have hurt you. We will try to be better parents."

That conversation led to many more about the whole situation and opened the door for us to discuss many sexual subjects as our kids matured. Most of all, that initial conversation modeled to our kids that God is gracious. Even parents make mistakes, but God is forgiving and can heal people and marriages if they let him.

Throughout this book, I have encouraged you to tell your own stories. This would certainly include stories about your experience of God's grace in your life. No sin can separate us from the love of God. Your kids need to know this wonderful truth as they grow, learn, love, and sometimes fall during their journey.

Sometimes the task of parenting is simply to put our arms around our kids, say we love them, tell them to trust a Father who is perfect in ways we can't be, and ask them to hold on. If we are prayerfully trying to model how God's love works in marriage, this will be enough.

HEALTHY SEXUALITY CHECKLIST

A healthy child emerging from adolescence will demonstrate several qualities in accordance with our healthy sexuality model.

Physical. Children will like their body, feel that it is attractive, and nurture it. They will be fully aware of the process of human sexual response and problems that can develop.

Emotional. Children will be able to talk openly about their feelings and not try to avoid them or hide them in substance abuse or unhealthy behaviors. Parents will need to monitor their children for negative self-talk or depression.

Relational. Children will develop safe friendships of both genders, experiment with love and romance, and build a community of support. Parents will need to continue to set boundaries and help their children make wise decisions about the people they associate with.

Personal. Children will heal any painful wounds from earlier stages, find professional help to do so if necessary, know how to have safe boundaries for themselves in all aspects of their lives, and be comfortable with their sexuality. Parents will need to monitor their children for symptoms of unresolved trauma.

Spiritual. Children will build their own relationship with God, embrace a vision for their lives of spiritual *agape* love in a possible marital relationship, rely on the power of God, and learn how to accept God's grace.

This has been a hard chapter to digest, I'm sure. The teenage years are demanding, but loving parents will understand the hard work that is required to get through them. If you don't already have support, seek out other Christians who are parenting teens or whose kids have already passed through this stage. As you choose to get support, you will be modeling healthy Christian fellowship to your child. This is an extremely valuable lesson. Those teenagers who decide to choose abstinence before marriage will need support and accountability from others. I will discuss this further in the next chapter as we examine the issues facing young adults.

CHAPTER EIGHT

Young Adulthood

(A G E   2 0   A N D   B E Y O N D)

Zach, age twenty, was a sophomore at a state university. He was far away from home and came back only for holidays. He was struggling with grades but getting by. He had found a fraternity that he really liked. His parents had met some of his new friends and basically liked them.

Zach's parents didn't drink, and he didn't experiment with alcohol until he started going to fraternity parties. When he came home for Christmas that second year, his dad could tell that something was wrong. He asked Zach if he wanted to talk. Zach said, "Dad, I'm feeling really bad. At one of our recent frat parties, I got pretty blitzed. There was this girl there, we hit it off, and we went back to her dorm. I don't remember a lot of what happened, but when I woke up the next morning I was in bed with her."

Zach looked miserable, and his dad knew that the situation raised many topics for serious conversation: fraternities, drinking, sex, safety, and so on. For now, though, he knew what he needed to say first. "Son, that is really hard. I love you and I'm glad you could tell me. Something like that also happened to me in college. Would you like to hear about it?"

When your kids reach the age of twenty and beyond, they are obviously adults, and your role as a parent has changed. It is now possible for you to have more of a mutual relationship or friendship with your children. They have passed through each developmental stage and hopefully have accomplished the basic tasks of maturing in healthy ways. If they haven't, then certain developmental issues will be replayed throughout their lives until they resolve them.

As your children transition from adolescence into young adulthood, you will recall the years you watched them eat junk food, ignore sleep or sleep all day, dress like something from outer space, and treat their rooms like the city dump. You have had to effect the personality of the Gestapo to get them to eat something nutritious, dress respectfully for church, and discover the drawers in their rooms. Now they may be off to college or their own apartment, and you begin to notice some encouraging changes. Maturity is somehow making occasional appearances. It is amazing what transformations a little responsibility will prompt. And, if they have worked through earlier tasks, your children now are ready for true spiritual and emotional intimacy.

At this stage many young people are purposefully launching their search for a mate, if they haven't found one already. There seems to be a national trend to postpone this search for a few years, so the average age of first marriage has increased; but for most young people the quest is on. Careers are starting as well. The search for meaningful work begins during this time and continues for years to come. Spiritually, this is a time of discerning God's calling for their lives.

As parents of young adults, your primary task is to let go and be sure you are not trying to hold on to or control your kids. Your second task is to love and support them as best you can while still respecting them as adults who must be responsible for their own lives.

If the conversations you have had with your children throughout their lives have had their intended effect, your young adults will feel forever free to come to you with questions or problems about sexuality that may develop later in their lives. It may not be your job to assist directly with these problems, but you can listen and continue to provide wise counsel when it is sought. A young adult who has received appropriate modeling and instruction will not need to have new conversations about all of the bases we have covered so far, but he or she may need some gentle reminders and continued modeling of healthy sexuality. If problems with sexuality develop for your children as adults and they come to you for help, then help them find the best resources you can. Continue to model for them all the aspects of healthy sexuality we've discussed.

HEALTHY SEXUALITY DURING YOUNG ADULTHOOD: PHYSICAL DIMENSION

Most young adults feel a compelling need to look good. Being health conscious and learning how to take care of themselves may come rather naturally now (to their parents' relief!). For young people, this stage of life often involves a process of exploration to discover the true significance of treating the body as a temple because it houses God's Spirit.

However, if issues of not liking one's appearance are left over from adolescence, they will continue to manifest themselves in a variety of ways.

Maggie never really liked the way she looked. Throughout her teenage years and now in young adulthood, she continually changed her wardrobe and the way she wore her hair. Now at twenty-one, she has begun going to the health club a lot and continues to believe that she doesn't have a good enough figure. She dates, but all the men she spends much time with are overweight or unkempt.

Maggie's parents decided to sit down with their daughter and explore her feelings. It was apparent to them that she was still seeing herself as the "ugly duckling." She was surrounding herself with men who reflected in their appearance how she saw herself. Her dad took the lead.

"Maggie, maybe I haven't told you enough: You are a really attractive young woman. God has given you such a wonderful appearance. I wonder why you have such a hard time believing it yourself. How can I help you to know that? Can you tell me how you feel?"

Maggie may simply need to talk with other young women who share the same feelings. Parents can't underestimate the power of the support of others who experience the same emotions and problems. Her parents may be able to help her to find such support.

HEALTHY SEXUALITY DURING YOUNG ADULTHOOD: EMOTIONAL DIMENSION

Healthy development in the emotional dimension involves learning to be honest and vulnerable and accepting responsibility for one's actions rather than blaming others. Young people will continue their emotional development by being honest and having true intimacy with each other, including members of the opposite sex. By this time, hopefully, you will have already modeled talking about feelings and taking responsibility, so conversations with your adult children will only be a continuation of what has come before.

If your children have unresolved issues about using various substances or behaviors to avoid or change their feelings, the relative freedom of young adulthood may cause destructive or addictive behaviors to escalate. Smoking, drinking, or sexual acting-out may become a more serious problem now.

Young adults who have not learned in earlier stages to be honest about their feelings and to be intimate with others will have particular problems in relationships, especially marriage. Because they don't know how to be intimate, they may wrongly assume that sex, in marriage or outside of marriage, will meet all their needs for love, touch, and nurture. If they continue to substitute sex for intimacy, they will be perpetually disappointed in relationships. They will continue to experience the pain of finding out that sex, even with a marriage partner, doesn't cure the wounds of loneliness created by one's inability to connect emotionally. Loneliness, disillusionment, and anger may cause them to keep seeking the solution in ever more addictive or destructive sexual behaviors. Fantasy, masturbation, prostitution, pornography, extramarital affairs, or various aberrant behaviors may escalate during this time.

Marty came to his dad, Richard, in despair. He was facing bankruptcy. Marty's credit cards were maxed out, and he was in debt for $40,000. His dad asked him what he had spent all this money on. Marty simply replied that he couldn't say. His dad said, "Son, if we're going to help you out of this, I need to know. I need to make sure that this isn't a bailout, and I need to be certain that it won't happen again." Marty finally and painfully confessed that he had used his credit cards to make calls to phone-sex services, buy pornography, and hire prostitutes.

Richard knew that the time he had feared had come. He had seen signs of potentially destructive sexual behavior in Marty's youth. There were the occasional discoveries of pornography stashed in Marty's room. There was the phone call from the parent of one of Marty's girlfriends who said she overheard the two of them talking sexually over the phone. When Marty was young, Richard had been too ashamed of his own problems with sexual sin to do much about what he suspected. Now he had to.

Richard had had many of the same problems that Marty did. Recently he had found help through his pastor, who directed him to counseling and support groups for sex addicts. He had made tremendous progress over the past three years. Painfully, Richard told Marty his own story. He didn't want to; he was afraid that his own son wouldn't love or respect him anymore. But when he was finished, Marty fell into his dad's arms and said, "Dad, I love you. Please help me get the help you did."

This broken young man will find help because of his dad's courageous example of emotional health. Richard modeled intimacy by taking a risk and choosing to be vulnerable. Even though Richard was not able to do this well while his son was growing up, Marty, as a young adult in trouble, can learn from his dad now and find God's healing in his own life.

HEALTHY SEXUALITY DURING YOUNG ADULTHOOD: RELATIONAL DIMENSION

As young adults, our children will continue to learn the importance of friendships. They will realize that, in order for any of us to be the people we want to be in all areas of our life, including our sexuality, we need support and accountability.

Accountability

Nick was a college student whose dorm room had access to the Internet. One night he discovered that he could access all kinds of Web sites that had pornography on them. Night after night, he found himself visiting those sites. He knew that he needed to stop but had trouble doing so. From ten o'clock at night until two o'clock in the morning were the worst times. Practicing being vulnerable, Nick was honest with a few of his friends about the struggles he was having with pornography. He asked four of them if they would call or stop by his room during that time every night. All four of his friends confessed that they also struggled with sexual purity in various ways. These five young men formed an accountability group and helped to keep each other pure all through college.

I find that the story of Nehemiah in the Old Testament gives a rather striking picture of accountability in the face of giants, enemies, and dangers—the things Nick and his friends faced every day in early adulthood. Nehemiah was one of the Jews taken captive when a foreign power conquered Israel. He had a rather good, if potentially dangerous, job as cupbearer to King Artaxerxes of Babylon.

The story starts with Nehemiah becoming aware that the city of his ancestry, Jerusalem, is in ruins. Nehemiah was saddened by this news, and the king asked why he appeared downcast. He explained his sorrow, and the king granted his request to go home and rebuild the city. Nehemiah was emboldened by this and asked for materials and letters of reference. He needed these for safe passage.

Artaxerxes was a wise king and knew that Nehemiah would need the cavalry to go with him for protection. This is the first application for our young adults: You shouldn't go on a journey through dangerous territory alone. So it is with the journey of life. A young person, feeling rather independent, must be taught that the dangerous journey of life must be undertaken with the "cavalry" of other people.

When Nehemiah arrived in his hometown, he found the city nearly destroyed. Sometimes, when I look around at our current culture, I get the same feeling. Morally, many things lie in ruins, many walls have been torn down, many safe barriers have crumbled. Nehemiah was wise enough to ask for help in rebuilding, and he was confident that, together, he and his friends could achieve their goal:

> Then I said to them, "You see the trouble we are in: Jerusalem lies in ruins, and its gates have been burned with fire. Come, let us rebuild the wall of Jerusalem, and we will no longer be in disgrace." (Nehemiah 2:17)

Our young adults need to be continually encouraged to reach out to others for help as they try to live pure and productive lives. They also need to be reminded that when people try to build their lives for God, particularly if they seek to change damaging behaviors, there will be those who don't like it.

> But when Sanballat, Tobiah, the Arabs, the Ammonites and the men of Ashdod heard that the repairs to Jerusalem's walls had gone ahead and that the gaps were being closed, they were very angry. They all plotted together to come and fight against Jerusalem and stir up trouble against it. But we prayed to our God and posted a guard day and night to meet this threat. (Nehemiah 4:7-9)

As our young people try to lead moral lives, they may be attacked and undermined by other people, sometimes even by friends and family. The most powerful shield against these threats is prayer. Living a healthy life in all the dimensions takes a lot of work. It's easy to get tired. Nehemiah's plan to remain strong will work for all of us:

> Therefore I stationed some of the people behind the lowest points of the wall at the exposed places, posting them by families, with their swords, spears and bows. After I looked things over, I stood up and said to the nobles, the officials and the rest of the people, "Don't be afraid of them. Remember the Lord, who is great and awesome, and fight for your brothers, your sons and your daughters, your wives and your homes." (Nehemiah 4:13-14)

Nehemiah stationed the workers and the warriors as family units. Since Old Testament times, the strength of the family has been the main line of defense for God's people. Nehemiah's great battle cry urged the people to fight for their brothers, their sons and daughters, their wives, and their homes.

Young people need to recognize that their fight for sexual fidelity is for their brothers and sisters, their future spouses, and their future homes. They also need to know that accountability is not just about asking others to help us; it is also about committing ourselves to help others. We fight for them. In fact, sometimes we gain more strength by giving than we do by receiving. Young people should be challenged to fight for each other and also for their future family. They don't know how many children they will have or who their future spouse will be, but they need to fight for sexual fidelity today.

Nehemiah also reminds us that when we fight for each other, God will fight for us:

> Those who carried materials did their work with one hand and held a weapon in the other, and each of the builders wore his sword at his side as he worked. But the man who sounded the trumpet stayed with me.

Then I said to the nobles, the officials and the rest of the people, "The work is extensive and spread out, and we are widely separated from each other along the wall. Wherever you hear the sound of the trumpet, join us there. Our God will fight for us!" (Nehemiah 4:17-20)

The ultimate strategy for rebuilding Jerusalem's wall required the people to be on guard day and night and to build with one hand and carry a weapon with the other. Likewise, we should always be ready for the attack. Finally, we see that Nehemiah kept the trumpet player with him so he could sound the alarm at the weakest points. Most of us don't have trumpets, but we do have phones. Young people are good with phones; most of them have cellular phones and pagers these days. They should use them in times of trouble and danger.

The principles we learn from Nehemiah are some of the great principles of accountability:

- Never journey through life alone.
- Ask for help.
- There is strength in families.
- Prepare in times of strength for times of weakness.
- Always be on guard.
- Fight for others and you will strengthen yourself.
- God will fight for those who depend on him.

If young people can learn to practice these principles, they will be much better equipped to lead pure lives, both before and after their wedding day.

Healthy Friendship

I have noticed an encouraging trend among young people in our culture: They seem to be better than my generation was at being true friends, especially with the opposite sex. This is a very good thing, especially because the healthy sexuality model teaches that healthy marriage partners must be friends first. They will also have solid and intimate friendships outside of their marriage relationship. These friendships provide many things, including support and accountability. Considerable research demonstrates that marriages are much stronger if neither spouse depends solely on the other for all of their support.

If your young adult has successfully come through the earlier developmental stages, he or she will be independent, emotionally strong, and capable of participating in many healthy friendships—those in which both people can relate intimately without losing a sense of their own identity. Such healthy friendships are based on mutuality, reciprocity, and honesty— all critical building blocks in the foundation of a solid marriage.

One of the tests of whether or not a young couple is emotionally and spiritually mature is how they handle the question of sex when it comes up in their relationship. If one person is immature and believes that sex is a way of getting affirmation from the other, then the friendship still needs to mature. The same is true if one person believes that he or she must be sexual in order to maintain the affection and presence of the other.

Roxanne came to her mom and dad and said, "I don't know what to do. I really love my boyfriend, but he has me really confused. Bill says that he wants to marry me, and I think I want to marry him too. But he says that as long as we love each other and intend to be married, it is okay to have sex now. He is so demanding. He says he is really frustrated. A lot of other guys he knows are being sexual with their girlfriends. I don't want to lose him. What should I do?"

Roxanne's dad took the lead on this one, "Honey, Bill is a great guy. He is a neat young Christian man, and Mom and I think a lot of him. But I believe that he is misguided about sex, just like I was at his age. We have already talked some about this. You know that healthy sexual intimacy is something that a married couple develops over time. It is not something to be experimented with now, just to see how you do with each other or to 'prove' your love. If you truly love each other and do get married, sex will be even better if you've waited.

"I'm sure that Bill's sexual appetite is strong. You are a beautiful young woman. He needs to know that you expect him to value you as an emotional and spiritual partner first and then to honor God's design for sex in marriage. If he needs to talk about this with some other young men who are committed to sexual purity, our pastor can find him some. If he truly loves you, he will be willing to wait.

"I know that if you enforce what you believe, you risk losing him, but from Mom's and my perspective, it is worth the risk. Your mom had to calm me down a bit before we were married and, at the time, I didn't like it. But now I'm so glad we waited."

Even as I write this story, I can hear the cultural voices in the back of my head: "What an old-fashioned way to talk! What kind of a prude is this father? Why doesn't he get with the times?" But truth is truth, however old. Roxanne will have to make up her own mind.

Clearly, our child's young adulthood can be a difficult stage for parents. We may not always like our children's choice of friends or romantic partners, and it's tempting to voice all of our opinions and try to control their choices. Occasionally, when we see our kids involved in obviously destructive relationships, we must intervene; but generally, this is the stage in which we must truly let go, allowing them to make their own mistakes and to learn the unique lessons God has ordained for them.

Marriage and Beyond

Consider for a moment the normal developmental process involved in growing a healthy marriage. In the early days, just like babies, we don't know much (even if we think we do). Later, like children with a parent, we often develop an enmeshed relationship with the "love of our life," the only other person in the world. But then one day, like adolescents, we wake up and discover that something has changed. We realize we are different from our spouse. The old saying "The honeymoon is over" becomes startlingly true. One day we wake up next to our spouse and wonder, "Did I really marry him (or her)? This is not what I bargained for." Our disillusionment may be over minor things like her not putting the cap on the toothpaste or him leaving the toilet seat up, or it may be a more serious frustration over issues of sexual compatibility or emotional satisfaction. Whatever its source, this disillusionment is a normal part of most people's marital journeys. Like teenagers, we may go through periods when we experiment again with our individuality. But as we mature as adults, we recognize that we truly love our spouse despite some differences, and we hunker down for the rest of life. This is the ideal development.

Many couples get stuck in one of the early stages. I got a letter the other day from a wife who said that her husband seemed to pick fights every few weeks. Then there would be a dramatic reconciliation, flaming romance, and great sex. He seemed to be re-creating the early stages of marriage over and over again. Other couples get stuck in the stage of recognizing and focusing on differences. In our culture there is lots of "permission" to think that you married the wrong person and deserve to find the "right" one. This way of thinking leads to affairs and contributes to our society's outrageous divorce rate.

As parents, you should be aware of where you are in your own marriage and be available to talk with your adult children about their marital challenges when appropriate. Wise parents know that life is a process and that marriage is a journey. One of Satan's deceptions involves trying to convince us that we married the wrong person. While sometimes it is dangerous to remain in a marriage and leaving is necessary, we need to recognize that there is no perfect marriage. It is a lie to think that perfect couples exist and have no problems.

John and Barb had been married for several years. One child came along. Finances were tight and life was generally stressful. They found that they fought about money, sex, and who should take care of their baby. They were dumbfounded. It certainly wasn't like this while they were dating and on their honeymoon. John and Barb were despondent when they went home for Thanksgiving. Barb's mom noticed how tired her daughter was. John's dad saw in his eyes the strain of a young man trying to earn a living.

After having dinner together, these four wise parents sat their children down and said simply, "You guys are in one of the hardest stages of a marriage. We know that there are stresses and tensions. We also remember the joy of your early years and know that it has somehow gotten buried in a pile of diapers and bills. We know. We went through this stage. We used to argue about many things. Through it all maybe we were just too stubborn to quit. We continued to pray even when we didn't feel like it, and we spent some time in marriage counseling. It was the best thing we ever did. It is normal for you to be where you are. How can we help?"

Parents may wonder how to offer support without being too invasive with their children. There is certainly wisdom in discretion. Remember, however, that it is rarely a mistake to share your own experience, strength, and hope. You don't have to pry by asking specific questions about sex, money, or anything else. Simply offer your experience and help.

Sometimes your married children may come to you and ask specific questions.

Bob told his dad. "I don't know what to think, Dad. When Jan and I first got married, everything was fine. Now that our baby is here, she seems depressed a lot. She certainly doesn't want to have sex with me. I'm really frustrated."

Bob's dad said, "Your mom and I went through a stage like that when you were born. You know a woman goes through tremendous hormonal changes when she has a baby. Sometimes depression is part of that. Jan is a wonderful woman. She gave up a great career that she loved to stay home and be with the baby. She naturally misses doing something she loved. I know she loves the baby and is committed to her decisions, but I wonder if she feels trapped right now.

"Having a baby also changes a woman's body some. She may not like her appearance as much. With all the physical changes and the stress of being a new mother, I'm not surprised by what you're going through. Your job is to affirm her, not to be angry about a natural process that will take time to resolve itself. She is not rejecting you or the baby.

"When is the last time you told her how much you love her and how beautiful she is? When is the last time you told her about your commitment to her regardless of whether or not she has sex with you when you want it?"

Of course, our adult children may face much more serious problems.

Jeff came to his dad and said, "I'm really stupid. For the last six months I've been having an affair. Things were going so badly at home. Kathy was busy with the kids, and she didn't seem to have time for me. This woman at the office gave me so much attention and praise. Now I'm hooked into that relationship and don't know how to get out of it. I'm afraid that the woman will create problems at the office, and I still need to work with her. I don't know whether to tell Kathy or not. What should I do?"

Jeff's dad felt compassion for his son's pain, but he also called him to a higher spiritual plane. "I'm really glad that you came to me, Jeff. I understand how this happened. It sounds like you have been tormented for a long time. In part, that is your conscience telling you the affair is wrong. You and Kathy have a God-ordained and sacred relationship.

"The first thing that you need to do is stop the affair. No job is worth the consequences of continuing it. If you need help in knowing what to say, we'll talk that through. If you have to quit your job, you can survive. Mom and I will help as much as we can. You simply can't compare the excitement of this affair with committed married love that will last a lifetime. You may think that you love this other woman, but you're living in fantasy. It is not fair to Kathy. If this other woman is creating some problems or threats, you may have to face the consequences of that. Don't let your anxiety about what she might do prevent you from doing the right thing.

"I can't give you all of the answers about telling Kathy. You will need to get some

counseling about that. I do think that if you want to have genuine intimacy with her, you will need to tell her how lonely you have been. The two of you will need to get some help to bridge the distance in your marriage that you've both been experiencing. An affair is usually a symptom of deeper problems, and you will have to take the lead on bringing those problems out into the light. Then you will need to work on them together.

"If consequences result from your actions, you will have to explain them to Kathy. If you have exposed yourself to the remotest possibility of sexually transmitted disease, it is only fair that both of you get tested. The main thing is that you stop the affair. If you do decide to tell Kathy about it, it will be better to come to her in true repentance, having stopped the relationship.

"Son, all your life I have tried to teach you to do the honorable thing. I am not judging you. God knows that I have been dangerously close to having an affair a couple of times myself. The honorable thing now is to humbly seek to repair your marriage, to be a faithful husband and an available father.

"If you do tell Kathy, she will be hurt and angry, and her trust will be destroyed. She will need to get some support and counseling. Healing will take a long time. It will be between her and God to accomplish that. If you turn your life around, commit your marriage to Christ, and start doing the right thing, God will honor that and help both of you."

The healing journey of recovery from sexual sin in a marriage is a long one. But there is hope. My wife and I are testimony to that. As parents you may have to deal with a child's marital difficulties more than once. Your children may also encounter more serious sexual or domestic problems that involve legal, financial, physical, or social consequences. Don't try to "fix" these complex problems; encourage your children to get specialized help. Meanwhile, speak the truth in love. Challenge your adult children to repent of sinful behavior and continue to become the people God wants them to be. Offer as much support as you can in every way, but never back down from the truth of God's design for healthy sexuality.

HEALTHY SEXUALITY DURING YOUNG ADULTHOOD: PERSONAL DIMENSION

Unhealed Wounds

In young adulthood, any unhealed emotional or sexual wounds your children have from the past will affect how they feel about themselves and how they relate to others. Leftover shame may keep the "I am a bad and worthless person" tapes running in your adult child's head. I believe it is the ongoing task of parents to monitor their children's destructive thinking if it could lead to dangerous behavior, depression, or misery.

Sam, twenty-five, was a bright young man, doing well in his career, and married for one year to Sue. He and his dad were playing golf one day. His dad noticed that he wasn't his usual self and asked him if there was anything wrong. With a deep sigh, Sam said, "It's embarrassing to talk about." After a long pause he went on, "Sue is really frustrated with me." After another long pause Sam went on, "It's about sex. Don't get the wrong idea, Dad. I've been faithful, that's not the problem. I seem to have lost total interest, and I wasn't all that interested to start with. Sue is wondering if there is something wrong with her, and I'm wondering if there's something wrong with me. Sue is beautiful to me. I always have good intentions about making love, but when we get close, I totally shut down. I don't know what to do. I've got to be the only man who feels this way."

"Son, that must be tough," Sam's dad said. "I know that you're not the only man who feels this way." After a while his dad went on, "There's something I've never told you, but I think you need to hear it now. When I was a young boy, an older boy in my neighborhood forced me into being sexual with him. I was horrified, but he was bigger and I didn't know what to do. Fortunately, he never tried this again and eventually he moved away.

"I thought I forgot about it, but when mom and I got married, I found there were times when I was afraid of sex and turned off by it—not always, just sometimes. I really struggled, thinking I was different too. Mom talked me into seeing a Christian

counselor. In counseling, I started remembering things, including that boy. Well, this is too long a story for the golf course, but I'm willing to tell you more details if you want. The main thing is that my counselor had me meet with a group of men who struggled with various sexual issues like I did. I met many guys whom I love like brothers today. We all had stories like mine. What a relief it was. Mom had to be patient, but eventually God healed my memories and I haven't had a problem since. If you want, I can give you the name of the counselor I saw."

What a courageous father. You see again the power of telling your own story. Until he needed to help his son, he had considered this story to be between his wife and him, but now his honest sharing about his own sexual wounds may open the door for Sam to find healing. Sam may decide to see that counselor and explore some parts of his past. His story may not be the same as his dad's, but he does have a story. Sam's dad may not ever know his son's story, but my guess is that he will choose someday to tell his dad what the process of healing was like for him. This patient and wise father has passed on a great gift and a real legacy, one that can help break the chain of sexual problems or sin in future generations.

Maybe you don't have a story to tell like Sam's dad did, but you can still be supportive if your kids come to you with specific problems. Help them find people who do have similar stories or direct them to counselors who can help them find healing for their personal wounds.

HEALTHY SEXUALITY DURING YOUNG ADULTHOOD: SPIRITUAL DIMENSION

Rebellion

During a young adult's ongoing quest for independence, it is not uncommon for him or her to stray from church and personal dependence on God. A young person feels healthy, strong, productive. "Who needs God?" he or she might think. As with so many stages in a child's developmental process, it is hard for parents to stand back and watch as their child's pride and self-sufficiency lead him away from some of the values they hold dear.

A period of sexual experimentation and its possible consequences can be one result of a young adult's spiritual rebellion. Unfortunately, for some only the experience of life's harsher realities and consequences will convince them that they need God. A parent's role during this time is simply to gently affirm biblical values, model them, and be willing to talk when asked.

Bonnie and Bill, both in their fifties, were excited about their son Matthew's upcoming Christmas visit. He was bringing home his girlfriend, Carmen, and they were looking forward to meeting her. Bonnie got Matthew's old room ready. Matthew's younger sister was off to college, so Bonnie prepared that room for Carmen. When Matthew and Carmen arrived, Bonnie and Bill liked her right away. That evening, Matthew came to his dad and said, "There's something you need to know. Carmen and I have been living together. We intend to get married someday, but we're not ready yet. We both love our jobs, and we're concentrating on those right now."

Both Bonnie and Bill were stunned and disappointed by this news and struggled to refrain from preaching about their opinions. They stopped short of telling Matthew that they were disappointed and that they hoped he would continue to think this through and remember some of the teaching from his youth. The next morning, however, they were shocked to see Carmen nonchalantly coming out of Matthew's room in her bathrobe.

Bill took his son out for coffee while Bonnie and Carmen went shopping. "Son, I'm going to try not to preach to you. You know how I feel about God and his will for marriage. I accept that right now you don't agree with me on that. I do need you to know that Mom and I still have certain boundaries at our house. One of those is that only married people sleep together in it. I need you and Carmen to respect that boundary. Otherwise you'll have to stay at a motel."

This is a painful situation for any Christian parent. I think that these two parents handled it as well as possible. They didn't preach, yet they were honest about their values. They also honored biblical ideals in their home. If a young adult is treated respectfully like this, he or she will get the message. The modeling and teaching of Matthew's youth will be there for him when he is willing to consider it again. I know that when I was at the height of my sexual sin and rebellion against God, many godly voices and teachings went through my head, but I had to learn some lessons the hard way. God was in control and eventually showed me a way out. When I finally grabbed on to a lifeline that other adults offered me, the spiritual truths from my youth propelled me to repent.

Agape Love

The vision of a young person in relationship with a potential marriage partner should be about *agape,* the spiritual kind of love that exists in Christ. I met a young couple recently who told me how they were pursuing this kind of love.

"We know that the kind of love God intends for us is essentially a spiritual love that will last a lifetime. Right now we have a lot of physical and emotional feelings that attempt to distract us from that vision, so we begin each of our dates together with a prayer, asking God to help us, to keep us safe, to grow our love for each other, to show us ways to avoid getting into situations where the physical temptations are overwhelming. Of course we have erotic feelings for each other. We also recognize that when we are feeling very emotionally intimate, we really want to express that deep friendship sexually. That is why we know we need to be careful. We have other young couples that we talk to and have accountability with."

This young couple is on the right track. They are developing a spiritual relationship together. What a wonderful thing! They allow themselves to hold hands, to kiss, and so forth, but they recognize and agree on their boundaries. It is easy for young people to deceive themselves into thinking that they have more self-control than they do. All young couples need to talk to each other and prepare for safety, purity, and long-term fidelity.

Sacrifice

One of the most dangerous myths of our current culture is that sexual desire is uncontrollable and must be expressed. Myths like this speak to a person's selfish inclinations: "My needs are so important. My sexual desire is so powerful. What can I do?"

If a young person is to be sexually pure and spiritually mature, he or she must be willing to sacrifice selfish desires. Paul wrote to the Romans:

> Therefore, I urge you, brothers, in view of God's mercy, to offer
> your bodies as living sacrifices, holy and pleasing to God—this is
> your spiritual act of worship. Do not conform any longer to the
> pattern of this world, but be transformed by the renewing of your
> mind. Then you will be able to test and approve what God's will
> is—his good, pleasing and perfect will. (Romans 12:1-2)

In Paul's description of marriage in Ephesians 5 he compared the mystery of the union of "one flesh" to the relationship of Christ to the church. Christ died for the church. The vision that we should hold up to our young people is that they should be willing to "die" for each other, to sacrifice when necessary personal wishes and passions, including selfish sexual desires. Such sacrifice is a matter of spiritual growth and maturity and comprises one of the main tasks of this stage.

Paul's father knew that he was on fire with sexual desire. Paul's fiancée, Karen, was a beautiful young woman, and it was easy to understand Paul's attraction. Paul's dad took him out for coffee and had this conversation: "I don't want to embarrass you, Son. It is hard for any man to wait to be sexual until he's married. But I want to continue to challenge you with the noble calling of being a man of integrity and of honoring Karen. As Christian men, God asks us to be willing to sacrifice our selfish desires. This includes sexual ones. God also wants husbands to make a priority of protecting and loving our wives' bodies. In marriage, Karen will choose to share her body with you, and that will be a wonderful time. Right now you need to consider her body a treasure to protect. Many times in your mom's and my marriage, I've known it is my sacred duty to treat her with respect. I find that when I do that, she is so much more likely to be giving in return. It is one of those paradoxes of Christian faith: When we surrender ourselves, we get so much back."

Remember, a vision shows us something that's worth fighting for. It is not enough to simply tell our adolescents and young adults to stay sexually pure "because God said so." They know that God says so, but they want to know why. They are often willing to obey God, but they need a vision of what he is calling them to. Paul's dad reminded him of that vision. As parents you may play a vital role in your young adult's life, modeling and motivating him or her to continue fighting for the kind of godliness that's worth sacrificing for.

HEALTHY SEXUALITY CHECKLIST

As they enter adulthood and possible marriage, young adults should possess the following qualities.

Physical. Young adults should know how to take care of their bodies as temples of the Holy Spirit. They may need to continue to receive affirmation about their physical appearance if they have leftover issues of physical shame.

Emotional. Young adults should be fully able to express their feelings in the marriage relationship and in friendship. They should thoroughly deal with anything they have substituted for intimacy, including addictive behavior, so they can experience the authentic connection they need.

Relational. Young adults who choose to marry should start building that relationship. If they are married, they should practice principles of healthy communication with their spouse. All young adults should participate in community and develop relationships that can provide them with accountability.

Personal. Young adults should have already experienced healing of any trauma from the past and should pursue help if they have not. Such healing will mean that they are comfortable with themselves as sexual beings and as sexual partners in marriage.

Spiritual. Young adults should make their own decisions about their relationship with God while they continue to grow in their capacity for sacrifice and *agape* love in all their relationships, especially marriage.

Your journey as a parent will never really end, nor will your opportunities to influence your children in positive ways. Soon you may be going back to the early chapters of this book to remind yourself about the essentials of healthy conversation so you can be available to your grandchildren.

And so life goes on. Enjoy your unique and vital role as a parent. Celebrate the part you have been able to play in your children's healthy sexual development. Continue to welcome opportunities to model God's wonderful design.

A Vision for You

When my son Jon was learning to play golf, he exhibited some natural talent. He hit the ball powerfully, but it always hooked to the left. One day his grandfather, a skillful golfer, showed him how to hit it correctly. Sure enough, his shots went straight down the fairway. The next time we were out playing, Jon was back to hitting everything to the left. I asked him if he had forgotten what Grandpa had showed him. "No," he said. "Then why aren't you doing it?" I asked. "Because it doesn't feel comfortable, it hurts," he said.

Making changes in any area of life may not feel comfortable. If you have been silent about sexuality, you will feel uneasy becoming more talkative. Conversations may even be embarrassing and hurtful.

Jon needed lots of practice and more supervision until he got his golf stroke right. It still doesn't always work. In the conference championships his senior year in high school, he hit a shot out-of-bounds to the left and he missed the opportunity to go to the state tournament. It broke my heart as I saw that ball sail in the wrong direction.

Likewise, you will experience times of great joy as you practice new forms of communication with your children. But you also will encounter painful and awkward times. The key is to keep trying and practicing.

If your children don't always embrace the behavior you advocate, you may be tempted to think that it is your fault. The greatest parents I know are those who are able to admit their mistakes and seek to learn from them.

We serve a forgiving God, the only perfect Father there is. Don't forget that we are up against the world and the many negative influences of its current darkness. Also remember that nothing is impossible with God. Even if we have made serious mistakes, God is powerful enough to help us and our children come out whole on the other side. Trust the Spirit of God to intercede for you and your children in ways that you can't imagine.

> In the same way, the Spirit helps us in our weakness. We do not know what we ought to pray for, but the Spirit himself intercedes for us with groans that words cannot express. And he who searches our hearts knows the mind of the Spirit, because the Spirit intercedes for the saints in accordance with God's will.
>
> And we know that in all things God works for the good of those who love him, who have been called according to his purpose. (Romans 8:26-28)

I hope that you will also find human support for yourselves as parents. More and more I have become convinced that we parents need to talk to each other. We need to compare information and swap stories. If we communicate, we can find out what other parents are doing and what is working for them. This connection also allows us the opportunity to coordinate efforts, establish common boundaries, and monitor our children's behaviors.

More than anything, we need to know that we are not alone as we face the challenges of parenting. We need the support of other people who are coping with some of the same issues, and we need the accountability that community provides. As I have said, accountability is about intimate friendship and fellowship. It is about committing to the process and asking others to support us in doing so. I encourage you to find other couples to hold you accountable in talking to your children about sex through the years. You may find that you will make friends for life.

Sexuality can be such a wonderful part of the union between a husband and wife. Hopefully, with the help of your guidance, modeling, and instruction, your children will find that fulfillment. I have a vision for you, and I offer it in the form of a prayer:

God, may this reader's children one day come to their parents and say, "Thank you. Thank you for being there, for being an example, for taking time for me, for affirming me in times of strength, for drying my tears in times of weakness, for encouraging me, for disciplining me in love, for just talking. May I be as good a parent to my children as you were to me."

May God richly bless you.

Additional Resources

BOOKS

These books may provide you with more insight and practical help on the topics presented in this book:

The Wounded Heart by Dan B. Allender, Ph.D. This groundbreaking book on sexual abuse and recovery is published by NavPress.

How to Talk Confidently with Your Child About Sex by Lenore Buth. This Christian book is written from a biologically technical perspective. Part of a six-book series that presents technical information to kids at various stages, it is available from Concordia Publishing House.

Preparing for Adolescence by Dr. James Dobson. I have found this book from Tyndale helpful in addressing some technical and spiritual issues involved in this age range.

Kids on Line by Donna Rice Hughes and Pamela T. Campbell. Published by Revell, this book gives parents guidance on how to protect their children from the dangers of the Internet.

Faithful and True by Mark Laaser, Ph.D. This book about sexual addiction and sexual integrity is published by Zondervan. A companion workbook by the same title is published by Broadman & Holman.

Raising Sexually Pure Kids by Tim and Beverly LaHaye. This book, published by Multnomah, deals very specifically with biblical principles for marriage and sexuality.

What's Happening to Me? and *Where Did I Come From?* by Peter Mayle. These are the "picture" books I refer to for use with young children. Published by Carol Publishing, these books are illustrated in such a way that biological information is comprehensible to children ages four and up.

False Intimacy by Harry W. Schaumburg, Ph.D. This is another excellent resource on sexual addiction, published by NavPress.

HELPFUL ORGANIZATIONS

For help with sexual addiction, men, women, spouses, and teenagers can contact the Oasis Ministry of the Christian Alliance for Sexual Recovery: (601) 844-5128. This is a ministry that I work with and direct.

For general concerns including sexual issues, call the following organizations for referrals to counselors in your area:

- The American Association of Christian Counselors: (800) 526-8673
- Focus on the Family: (800) 232-6459
- New Life Treatment Centers: (800) 639-5433
- The National Coalition for the Protection of Children and Families: (513) 521-6227

For help with the fight against pornography, contact the American Family Association: (800) 326-4543.

Phone numbers sometimes change, so don't be frustrated if any of these are no longer in service. Call my office at (612) 949-3478 for the latest information about whom to contact for help.

Subject Index

About the Author

Mark R. Laaser, Ph.D., graduated from Princeton Theological Seminary with a degree in ministry and from the University of Iowa with a Ph.D. in pastoral counseling. He was a member of the National Council for Sexual Addiction/Compulsivity and currently serves on the Overcomer's Outreach and Interfaith Sexual Trauma Institute Boards. Dr. Laaser has designed programs for both inpatient and outpatient treatment of sexual addiction and has served as a consultant to the American Family Association, helping men and women struggling with pornography and other addictions. He has worked with several hundred pastors who have had problems with sexual sin and consulted with a wide variety of denominations and churches.

Dr. Laaser has lectured and conducted workshops about addictions, families, and marriage building around the country. He has also worked with Youth With A Mission, training missionaries to set up addiction-recovery programs in other parts of the world. He has written numerous articles for both academic journals and popular magazines, and he is the author or coauthor of several books including *Faithful and True, Before the Fall,* and *Restoring the Soul of a Church.* He is a frequent guest on radio and television. He lives in Minnesota with his wife, Deb, and their three children, Sarah, Jon, and Ben.